The Ketogenic Diet for Beginners

The Perfect Guide to Living a Keto-lifestyle with 120 High Fat, Low Carbs Recipes for Weight Loss

By Janie Lorrance

© **Copyright 2017 by Janie Lorrance**

All rights reserved.

This document is geared towards providing exact and reliable information in regards to the topic and issue covered. The publication is sold with the idea that the publisher is not required to render accounting, officially permitted, or otherwise, qualified services. If advice is necessary, legal or professional, a practiced individual in the profession should be ordered.

From a Declaration of Principles which was accepted and approved equally by a Committee of the American Bar Association and a Committee of Publishers and Associations.

In no way is it legal to reproduce, duplicate, or transmit any part of this document in either electronic means or in printed format. Recording of this publication is strictly prohibited and any storage of this document is not allowed unless with written permission from the publisher. All rights reserved.

The information provided herein is stated to be truthful and consistent, in that any liability, in terms of inattention or otherwise, by any usage or abuse of any policies, processes, or directions contained within is the solitary and utter responsibility of the recipient reader. Under no circumstances will any legal responsibility or blame be held against the publisher for any reparation, damages, or monetary loss due to the information herein, either directly or indirectly.

Respective authors own all copyrights not held by the publisher.

Table of Contents

Chapter One: Understanding the Ketogenic Diet............... 1
    What is the Ketogenic Diet?............................ 2
    Fuel Metabolism with the Ketogenic Diet................ 2
    How Does it Work?...................................... 3
    The Health Benefits of the Ketogenic Diet.............. 6

Chapter Two: Go to Start with Ketogenic Diet............... 11
    How to Get Started with Ketogenic Diet................ 12
    The Ketogenic Diet and Workouts....................... 14
    The Shopping List for the Ketogenic Diet.............. 16
    Recommended Food on Ketogenic Diet.................... 19
    Helpful Tips for the Ketogenic Diet................... 24

Chapter Three: The Ketogenic Diet Recipes................. 28
    The Breakfast Recipes................................. 29
        1. Healthy Smoked Salmon Omelet................... 29
        2. Healthy Green Omelet........................... 30
        3. Smoked Salmon & Red Pepper Scramble............ 31
        4. Healthy Frittata w/ Scallions & Smoked Salmon...... 32
        5. Yummy Super food Porridge...................... 33
        6. Spiced Salmon Frittata......................... 34
        7. Spicy Mexican Breakfast Scramble............... 36

8. Yummy Zucchini & Beef Frittata..................................37

9. Detoxifying Rainbow Acai Bowl..................................38

10. Choco Peanut Butter Milkshake................................39

11. Superfood Fruity Parfait..40

12. Delicious Breakfast Turkey Casserole.......................41

13. Spicy Breakfast Scrambled Eggs..............................42

14. Vegetable Breakfast Casserole................................43

15. Tasty Berry Omelet...45

16. Sausage & Broccoli Breakfast Quiche......................46

17. Avocado Shrimp Omelet..47

18. Yummy Breakfast Stir Fry..48

19. Tasty Breakfast Wrap..49

20. Chocolate Pecan Smoothie.....................................50

The Lunch Recipes..51

21. Satisfying Turkey Lettuce Wraps..............................51

22. Grilled Steak Salad w/ Buttermilk-Avocado Buttermilk Dressing..53

23. Lentil Coconut Curry Soup......................................54

24. Steamed Salmon w/ Fennel & Fresh Herbs............56

25. Fried Tofu w/ Spring Greens...................................57

26. Cashews-and Pretzel-Crusted Tofu........................58

27. Teriyaki Fish w/ Zucchini..60

28. Italian Fish Stew...61

29. Grilled Tuna w/ Bean & Tomato Salad....................62

30. Steamed Bass with Fennel, Parsley, and Capers......63

31. Turkey & Coconut Soup..64

32. Crunchy Kale & Almond Salad with Roasted Chicken 66

33. Chicken w/Red Onions & Kale 67

34. Tasty Chicken Greek Salad..69

35. Spiced Turkey Served with Avocado Relish........... 70

36. Yummy Seafood Salad..72

37. Chicken with Greek Salad...73

38. Chicken w/ Spicy Cauliflower Couscous.................. 74

39. Salmon w/ celery Salad, Rocket & Caramelized Chicory.. 76

40. Grilled Sardines w/ Wilted Arugula........................ 77

41. Healthy Salmon Super Salad..................................... 79

42. Fish w/ Olives, Tomatoes & Capers..........................80

43. Healthy Chicken Curry..81

44. Healthy Chicken Super Salad..................................... 82

45. Salmon Salad in Avocado Cups................................. 83

46. Beef Shred Salad..85

47. Delicious Baked Tilapia in Garlic & Olive Oil.......... 86

48. Tilapia with Herbs...87

49. Marinara Chicken..88

50. Lemon Garlic Salmon..89

The Dinner Recipes..90

51. Gingery Roasted Chicken......................................90

52. Tangerine Ham with Baby Carrots........................ 91

53. Pepper Crusted Steak...93

54. Tasty Sesame Salmon.. 93

55. Buffalo Chicken Fingers..95

56. Tasty Baked Chicken..96

57. Tasty Grilled salmon.. 96

58. Spiced Chicken Patties...98

59. Scrumptious Shrimp.. 99

60. Ground Beef Tacos... 100

61. Poached Halibut... 101

62. Crock Pot Coconut Curry Shrimp........................102

63. Beef Stir Fry w/ Red Onions & Peppers................ 103

64. Ginger Chicken with Veggies...............................104

65. Chili Fried Steak with Toasted Cashews............. 105

66. Tasty Coconut Cod 106

67. Grilled Chicken with Fresh Herb Marinade 108

68. Orange-Cranberry Crusted Salmon 109

69. Grilled Chicken & Green Onion 110

70. Shrimp Salad w/ Grapefruit and Avocado 111

71. Chicken Stir-Fry 112

72. Chicken and Mushroom Stew 113

73. Bacon, Beef Sausage and Broccoli Casserole 115

74. Herbed London Broil 116

75. Tasty Oregano Chicken 117

76. Tasty Citric Chicken 118

77. Healthy Stuffed Mushrooms 119

The Snacks Recipes 120

78. Roasted Chili-Vinegar Peanuts 120

79. Tahini Hummus 121

80. Baked Beet Chips with Tzatziki 122

81. Dry-Roasted Chickpea 124

82. Bacon-Avocado stuffed Peppers 125

83. Healthy Seed Crackers (Nut-Free, Vegan, Vegetarian, Gluten-Free) 126

84. Tasty Candied Pecans 127

85. Raw Protein-Packed Quinoa Energy Bars (Vegan, Vegetarian, Gluten-Free) 128

86. Healthy Roasted pumpkin seeds 129

87. Candied Macadamia Nuts 130

88. Barbequed Peaches & Plum with Cream Cheese .. 130

89. Healthy Spinach Cake 132

90. Grilled Pineapple Sundaes with Shredded Coconut 133

91. Vinegar & Salt Kale Chips 134

92. Minty Cucumber Popsicles 135

The Dessert and Drink Recipes 137

93. Green Tea Avocado Shake 137

94. Berry Power Shake 137

95. Superfood Chia Pudding 138

96. Healthy Berry Ice Cream 139

97. Delicious Berry Smoothie 140

98. Delicious Strawberry Punch 141

99. Almond-Strawberry Smoothie 142

100. Coconut- Coffee smoothie 143

101. Citrus Punch 144

102. Gingery Lemonade 145

103. Berry-Spinach Smoothie 146

104. Lime Lemon Slush...147

105. Slimming Smoothie...147

106. Gingery Grape Juice.. 148

107. Fat-Burner Juice..149

108. Garlicky Green Juice..150

109. Strawberry Coconut Milk Smoothie......150

110. Avocado-Raspberry Smoothie................151

111. Healthy Green Smoothie...152

112. The Super-8 Detox Juice...................................... 153

113. Sugar-Free Peanut Butter Protein Smoothie......154

114. Kale-Beetroot Juice.. 155

115. Ginger Spice Smoothie..156

116. Lemon Blueberry Bliss....................................... 157

117. Yummy Cinnamon Smoothie................................. 158

118. Mint-Infused Green Smoothie.............................159

119. Gingery Pineapple Paradise................................. 160

120. Toasted Coconut & Strawberry Smoothie.......... 161

Chapter One

Understanding the Ketogenic Diet

What is the Ketogenic Diet?

The ketogenic diet causes ketone bodies to be produced by your liver, thus shifting your body's metabolism away from using glucose as the primary source of fuel and toward fat utilization.

To accomplish this, the ketogenic diet restricts carbohydrate intake below a certain level – usually 100 grams per day. The daily amount depends on your health and weight loss goals.

Fuel Metabolism with the Ketogenic Diet

Free Fatty Acids (FFA) are one of the fuels that can be used for almost all tissues in your body. However, organs like your brain and nervous system cannot utilize FFA, but they can use ketone bodies.

Ketone bodies are byproducts of the incomplete breakdown of FFA in your liver, and they serve as a non carb, fat derived fuel for your brain and nervous system.

When the production of ketone bodies is accelerated, they accumulate in your bloodstream and develop a metabolic state known as ketosis. At the same time, there is a decrease in glucose production and utilization. Additionally, there is also a decrease in the breakdown of protein to be utilized as an energy source which is called protein sparing.

Many people looking to lose fat are drawn to the ketogenic diet because it allows for fat loss while sparing the loss of lean body mass, leaving you slim and toned.

How Does it Work?

We all know that we need food for energy. On a typical high-carb diet, your body specifically uses glucose as the primary source of energy. It is easier for your body to convert carbs to glucose than it is with other types of energy sources. Insulin will also be produced to process the glucose in your blood stream, and the fats will just be stored and will eventually pile up.

The ketogenic diet enables your body to use another energy source for fuel.

The concept is that with a lower carb intake, you will be depriving your body of the glucose it needs and will make use of the fats instead, as it falls into a state known as ketosis.

Ketosis is a natural state of the body wherein the liver will breakdown the available fats instead of glucose or carbohydrates, and ketones will be produced, which will be burned by the body as the energy source.

Your goal with the ketogenic diet is to force your body into this metabolic state. Your body is designed to easily adapt to a metabolic state, so you only need to worry about following the diet and let your body handle the rest.

The ketogenic diet is different from other low-carb diets. The difference is that your diet should be about 70-75 percent of calories from fat, 20-25 percent from protein, and 5-10 percent from carbohydrates each day. If you follow these guidelines, your diet will be composed of high-fats and moderate protein intake and there will be no need to count calories.

Protein is limited because it affects the insulin and blood sugar in your body. If you consume protein in large quantities, the excess gets converted to glucose. As a result, your body will not reach a state of ketosis.

Have you ever noticed that whenever you have a food craving, you usually go for carb-rich foods? That's because your brain has labeled the starchy and sweet foods as comfort foods. Our main goal with the ketogenic diet is to drastically reduce this sinful food category and choose a healthier alternative. In theory, if you limit your carb intake and achieve a state of ketosis, the excess weight will shed easily.

The Health Benefits of the Ketogenic Diet

Kills your appetite in a healthy way.

Hunger and deprivation are the worst side effects of any diet, and this is one of the main reasons why most diets fail. But not the keto diet. By cutting carbs and replacing them with healthy fats and protein, your body will take more time to digest fats and proteins than it did carbs and you will naturally eat less. In the end, you'll stay full longer and lose more weight!

Faster and sustainable weight loss

Cutting carbs is the fastest and surest way to quickly lose weight. First, a low-carb diet, such as the ketogenic diet, gets rid of all the excess water from your body. The first thing you will notice is the loss of water weight. Additionally, since the keto diet lowers your insulin levels, your kidneys start shedding the excess sodium which leads to rapid weight loss within the first two weeks.

For as long as you remain committed to the ketogenic diet, you will continue losing weight until you achieved your ideal weight.

Slimmer waist lines

Not all the fat in your body is the same. Where the fat is stored in your body is what will determine how your weight affects your health. There is subcutaneous fat which is stored under the skin and visceral fat that is stored within your abdominal cavity.

Visceral fat is dangerous because it tends to lodge around your organs. Fat around your abdomen can fuel insulin resistance and inflammation, and is believed to be the leading cause of chronic illnesses.

The ketogenic diet is very effective at reducing visceral fat and you will notice your waistline shrinking when you start following the ketogenic diet.

Increased levels of good cholesterol

Good cholesterol is biologically referred to as High Density Lipoprotein (HDL). Good cholesterol levels tend to increase under the ketogenic diet as your body carries the Low Density Lipoprotein (LDL) or the bad cholesterol away from your body and into the liver where it is recycled and excreted as waste.

Reduced symptoms of type 2 diabetes

When you eat a lot of carbs, your body breaks them down into simple sugars. Once this glucose gets into your blood stream, it elevates your blood sugar levels and triggers the release of insulin. The release of insulin instructs your cells to take in the glucose and use it, or store it as fat for later use.

Continued intake of low quality carbs, such as white bread or sweetened beverages, can lead to insulin resistance. When this happens, your cells are not able to recognize insulin and it becomes harder for your body to take the blood sugar into your cells. This is what leads to type 2 diabetes.

The only way to reverse this cycle is to cut carbs from your diet to the point where your body doesn't need to release high amounts of insulin.

In a scientific study of patients with type 2 diabetes, 95.2 percent of the patients were able to reduce or eliminate the use of their diabetes medication within six months of beginning the ketogenic diet.

However, if you are using medication, ensure you consult with your doctor to prevent incidences of hypoglycemia.

The ketogenic diet is therapeutic for several brain disorders

Did you know that there is a part of your brain that only burns glucose? When you cut out carbs, glucose is reduced, and as a result, your liver will produce glucose out of protein. However, there's a larger part of your brain that can burn ketones. Ketones are formed when you cut out carbs from your diet or are starving.

This process is the reason why the keto diet has been used to treat children with epilepsy who don't respond to medication. Additionally, the ketogenic diet has also been shown to reduce symptoms and prevent Alzheimer's disease, Parkinson's disease, and dementia, as well as improve cognitive function in general.

It's evident that with the ketogenic diet, it's a win-win situation for weight loss and a host other health benefits.

Chapter Two

Go to Start with Ketogenic Diet

How to Get Started with Ketogenic Diet

As you now know, the goal of the ketogenic diet is to allow your body to enter ketosis; but the question now is, how?

The ketogenic diet is categorized into three types –the Standard Ketogenic Diet (SKD), Targeted Ketogenic Diet (TKD), and Cyclical Ketogenic Diet (CKD). People who have sedentary lifestyles and wish to lose weight through a keto diet is advised to follow the SKD.

This diet recommends limiting the consumption of your carbs to 20-50 grams daily, which means your macros should be made up of 70-75 percent fat, 20-25 percent protein, and 5-10 percent carbs. The number of daily calories you can consume relies on your weight, height, age, and activity level. If you're unsure how to do this, you can always consult a keto calculator (click here).

You might be skeptical about the ketogenic diet right now, especially if you think that consuming less carbs will make you hungry. If you consume a healthy number of calories and eat foods that are nutrient dense (e.g. vegetables and healthy fats), then you don't have to worry about going hungry at all! When you do this, you can safely enter a state of ketosis.

However, unlike any other diets, the keto diet needs your complete commitment for you to achieve a state of ketosis. Depending on your body type, activity level, and your choice of macros, you can enter into ketosis anytime from two days to a week.

For beginners, it is advisable that you use urine ketone sticks (such as Ketosis) to monitor the levels of ketones in your body and ensure that you are in ketosis state. This is a useful tip to help you know whether your body is under ketosis and is burning fat as energy.

I must advise you however that before anything else, it is a must that you ask for a green light from your health care provider if you are planning to follow the ketogenic diet or any type of diet. Although this diet is safe, even for children, you must let your doctor know about this, especially if you have existing health conditions.

Pregnant women or those who are breast-feeding are not encouraged to try the ketogenic diet for weight loss because this may have adverse effects on their baby.

The Ketogenic Diet and Workouts

As with any diet with the goal of losing fat, exercise improves the efficiency and success of the ketogenic diet. However, it's important to note that when you eliminate carbs, your body cannot sustain high intensity exercises. Your best option is to do low intensity cardio exercises.

For this reason, if you are looking to make exercise a huge part of your ketogenic diet, you should integrate carbs without disrupting the ketosis process.

There are two types of modified ketogenic diets: Targeted Ketogenic Diet (TKD), which allows you to consume carbs before you exercise to sustain performance without impacting ketosis.

The Cyclical Ketogenic Diet (CKD) alternate periods of high-carb consumption with periods of ketogenic dieting. The cycle of high-carb consumption is aimed at refilling your muscle glycogen to sustain your workout.

The Shopping List for the Ketogenic Diet

Fruits

Raspberries, blueberries, strawberries, grapefruit, dates, cranberries, lemons, limes, navel oranges, avocados, currants, apples, and red grapes

Veggies

Garlic, plum tomatoes, scallions, mushrooms, ginger root, celery, red onions, romaine lettuce, cauliflower, broccoli, tomatoes, cucumber, cherry tomatoes, spinach, Kalamata, olives, beets, English cucumbers, green beans, zucchini, red pepper, kale, collards, carrots, shallots, and birds eye chili

Nuts & Seeds

Sunflower seeds, almond meal, pecans, almonds, pumpkin seeds, pine nuts, walnuts, natural peanut butter, sunflower seeds, poppy seeds, sesame seeds, silvered almonds, mustard seeds, macadamia nuts

Grains

wheat germ, oats, whole-wheat bread, buckwheat, quinoa, canned beans

Meats, Poultry, Fish & Seafood

Eggs, smoked salmon, capers, turkey, tuna steaks, salmon fillets, boneless chicken breasts, tilapia fillets, canned wild salmon, beef, bacon, ham, and halibut

Herbs and Spices

Cinnamon powder, garlic powder, fresh dill, red pepper flakes, fresh tarragon, fresh basil, parsley, turmeric, ground cumin seed, paprika, pickling spice, fennel fronds, chives, and ground pepper

Extras

Greek yogurt, almond milk, rapeseed oil, cottage cheese, extra-virgin olive oil, matcha, green tea, salt, maple syrup, desiccated coconut, protein powder, kosher salt, black olive tapenade, coconut flakes, coconut oil, pumpkin pie spice, pumpkin puree, mustard, raw honey, Dijon mustard, coarse grain mustard, white wine vinegar, balsamic vinegar, Worcestershire sauce, apple cider vinegar, sea salt, and diet ginger ale

Recommended Food on Ketogenic Diet

Fats and Oils

Because fats will make up most of your meals, you must choose the good type of fat that comes from natural sources, and avoid those that are dangerous to your health. Some of your best choices for fat are:

- Ghee or Clarified butter
- Avocado
- Coconut Oil
- Red Palm Oil
- Butter
- Coconut Butter
- Peanut Butter
- Chicken Fat
- Beef Tallow
- Non hydrogenated Lard
- Macadamia Nuts
- Egg Yolks

- Fish rich in Omega-3 Fatty Acids like salmon, mackerel, trout, tuna, and even shell fish.

Protein

To achieve a state of ketosis, you need to consume 20-25 percent of protein as part of your daily caloric allowance. This means your consumption of fat will be high, carbs are low, and protein is moderate. Of course, you also want to choose the healthy sources of protein that are either organic or grass fed.

- Meat— beef, veal, lamb, chicken, duck, pheasant, pork chops, pork loin, etc.
- Deli Meat— bacon, sausage, ham (make sure to watch out of added sugar and other fillers)
- Eggs— preferably free-range or organic eggs
- Fish— wild caught salmon, catfish, halibut, trout, tuna, etc.
- Seafood— lobster, crab, oyster, clams, mussels, etc.
- Peanut Butter—this is a great source of protein, but make sure to choose the all-natural variant

Dairy

Compared to other weight loss diets, the ketogenic diet actually encourages you to choose dairy products that are full fat. Some of the best dairy products that you can choose are:

- Hard and soft cheese— cream cheese, mozzarella, cheddar, etc.
- Cottage cheese
- Heavy whipping cream
- Sour cream
- Full-fat yogurt

Vegetables

Overall, vegetables are rich in vitamins and minerals that contribute to a healthy body. However, if you're aiming to avoid carbs, it's best that you keep away from starchy vegetables such as potatoes, yams, peas, corn, beans, and legumes. You also want to limit vegetables that taste sweet such as carrots and squash. Instead, stick with green leafy vegetables that are preferably organically grown and other low-carb veggies.

- Spinach
- Lettuce
- Collard greens
- Mustard greens
- Bok choi
- Kale
- Alfalfa sprouts
- Celery
- Tomato
- Broccoli
- Cauliflower

eat occasionally

Fruits

Your choice of fruit is only limited to avocado and some berries because fruits are high in carbs and sugar.

Drinks

- Water
- Black coffee
- Herbal tea
- Wine—white wine and dry red wine are OK if they are only consumed occasionally.

Others

- Homemade mayo—if you want to buy mayo from the store, make sure that you watch out for the carbs it contains
- Homemade mustard
- Any type of spices and herbs
- Honey
- Stevia
- Agave Nectar
- Ketchup (Sugar-free)
- Dark chocolate/cocoa

Helpful Tips for the Ketogenic Diet

Learn to Count Your Net Carbs— As you now know, the key to entering a state of ketosis is to limit your carbs to 20-25 grams of net carbs every day. One of the useful tools to help you monitor this is using an app called MyFitnessPal that can be downloaded on your device for free. With this app, you can easily log your foods and monitor the nutritional value of foods you consume.

Although this app doesn't provide you with your consumption of net carbs, it will provide you with the amount of fiber and carbs that you consumed. To get your net carbs, just simply subtract the fiber from the carbs you consumed.

Beware of Hidden Carbs— It will be very easy for you to avoid foods such as pastas and bread because you know that they are loaded with carbs. However, most people fail to count carbs that are hidden in foods such as baked beans, salad dressing, and tomato sauce which all have carbs in them. Make sure to read labels and count all carbs to stick to the 20-25 grams daily and achieve ketosis.

Choose the Right Foods— Even if the ketogenic diet is a low-carb, high-fat diet, this doesn't give you the liberty to consume as much fat as you can. Of course, you want the food you consume to be of quality and are rich in nutrients. But one good tip to remember is to just stay away from carbs such as pastas, breads, rice, and even sugar. The 20-25 grams of carbs that you're allowed to consume also includes the carbs from vegetables.

Limit Your Consumption of Fruit— Fruits have loads of vitamins, fiber, and other nutrients that are good for the body. However, if you want to reset your metabolism and allow it to use fat as fuel instead of glucose, then you must keep your consumption of fruit to a minimum. That's because all fruits are high in fructose, a type of sugar found in fruit, which causes your insulin levels to spike. When that happens, the fats cells in your body are locked and your body will use glucose as energy.

Remember that while following the ketogenic diet, you are only allowed to have 20-25 grams of net carbs a day. A medium-sized banana already amounts to 24 grams net carbs, which means, you almost have already consumed all your carbs for the day by eating one banana. If you still want to consume fruits, you can stick with a cup of mixed berries that has 5 grams of net carbs, but this is not recommended to be consumed daily.

Spend More Time in the Kitchen— For you to achieve ketosis, it is vital that you monitor all the food you eat. That's why it is advisable to prepare your own meals and avoid eating out too much. You will have to sacrifice a bit of your time in preparing your meals, but this assures you that you're only consuming what is approved in the ketogenic diet.

I've provided you with a list of recipes from breakfast to dinner in the next chapters to help you whip up your own keto approved meals in your kitchen. If you're ready to get started, turn the page now!

Chapter Three
The Ketogenic Diet Recipes

The Breakfast Recipes

1. Healthy Smoked Salmon Omelet

Yield: 1 Servings

Total Time: 20 Minutes

Prep Time: 10 Minutes

Cook Time: 10 Minutes

Ingredients

- 1 tsp. extra virgin olive oil
- 100 g sliced smoked salmon
- 1/2 tsp. capers
- 2 large eggs
- 10g chopped rocket
- 1 tsp. chopped parsley

Directions

1. Beat the eggs into a large bowl; stir in salmon, rocket, capers, and chopped parsley.

2. Add extra virgin olive oil to a nonstick pan and heat over medium heat until hot, but not smoking; add the egg mixture and spread the mixture evenly in the pan. Lower heat and cook until the omelet is cooked through.

3. With a spatula, roll up the omelet in half and serve hot.

Nutritional Information Per Serving

Calories: 303; Total Fat: 19 g; Carbs: 1.3 g; Dietary fiber: trace; Sugars: 1 g; Protein: 31.2 g; Cholesterol: 395 mg; Sodium: 2186 mg

2. Healthy Green Omelet

Yield: 1 Serving

Total Time: 20 Minutes

Prep Time: 10 Minutes

Cook Time: 10 Minutes

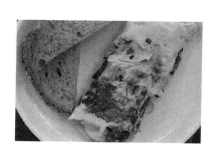

Ingredients

- 1 tsp. extra virgin olive oil
- 2 large eggs
- 1 red onion, finely chopped
- 2 tsp. chopped parsley
- Handful rocket leaves
- Salt and pepper

Directions

1. Heat oil in a frying pan set over medium low heat; stir in the red onion and fry for about 5 minutes. Cook over medium heat for about 2 minutes.

2. Whisk the eggs well and add to the pan with the onion; evenly distribute the egg mixture and cook for about 1 minute.

3. Lift the sides of the omelet to allow the uncooked egg slip in the base of the frying pan. Cook to your desired doneness and sprinkle with parsley and rocket.

4. Season with salt and pepper and roll up the omelet.

Serve right away.

Nutritional Information Per Serving

Calories: 228; Total Fat: 14.7 g; Carbs: 11.3 g; Dietary fiber: 2.5 g; Sugars: 5.4 g; Protein: 13.9 g; Cholesterol: 372 mg; Sodium: 146 mg

3. Smoked Salmon & Red Pepper Scramble

Yield: 1 Serving

Total Time: 15 Minutes

Prep Time: 10 Minutes

Cook Time: 5 Minutes

Ingredients

- 2 whole eggs and 1 egg yolk
- ⅛ teaspoon garlic powder
- 1 tablespoon chopped fresh dill
- 2 pieces smoked salmon, torn apart
- ⅛ teaspoon red pepper flakes
- Salt and pepper
- 1 tablespoon extra-virgin olive oil

Directions

1. Beat the eggs in a bowl; stir in garlic, dill, salmon, red pepper flakes, black pepper and salt until well combined.

2. Set a saucepan over low heat; add extra virgin olive oil. Once warm, add the egg mixture and cook, stirring until cooked through. Serve topped with roasted veggies.

Nutritional Information per Serving:

Calories: 376; Total Fat: 29.9 g; Carbs: 3.5 g; Dietary Fiber: 0.5 g; Protein: 24.9 g; Cholesterol: 550 mg; Sodium: 1272 mg; Sugars: 0.9 g

4. Healthy Frittata w/ Scallions & Smoked Salmon

Yield: 6 servings

Total Time: 30 Minutes

Prep Time: 10 Minutes

Cook Time: 20 Minutes

Ingredients

- 2 teaspoons extra-virgin olive oil
- 6 scallions, trimmed and chopped
- ½ teaspoon finely chopped fresh tarragon
- 2 ounces smoked salmon, sliced into small pieces
- 2 tablespoons black olive tapenade
- 4 large eggs
- 6 large egg whites
- ¼ cup water
- ½ teaspoon salt

Directions

1. Preheat your oven to 350°F.

2. Set a large ovenproof pan over medium heat; add oil and heat until hot, but not smoky. Stir in scallions and sauté, stirring, for about 3 minutes or until tender and fragrant.

3.In a bowl, beat together eggs, egg whites, tarragon, water, and salt; season with black pepper and pour into the pan.

4.Arrange the salmon onto the egg mixture. Cook, stirring frequently, for about 2 minutes or until almost set; transfer to the oven and cook for about 14 minutes or until puffed and golden.

5.Remove the frittata from the oven and transfer to a serving plate; slice and serve with tapenade.

Nutritional Information per Serving:

Calories: 186; Total Fat: 5 g; Carbs: 1 g; Dietary Fiber: trace; Protein: 10 g; Cholesterol: 143 mg; Sodium: 535 mg; Sugars: trace

5. Yummy Super food Porridge

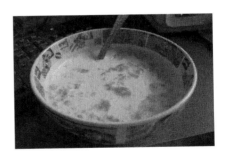

Yield: 4 Servings

Total Time: 20 Minutes

Prep Time: 10 Minutes

Cook Time: 10 Minutes

Ingredients

- 1½ cups almond milk
- Handful chopped almonds or walnuts
- 2 tablespoon ground flaxseed
- 3 tablespoon chia seeds
- 3 tablespoon shredded unsweetened coconut
- 1 teaspoon pure vanilla extract

- 1 scoop protein powder

Toppings:

- 1 tablespoon peanut butter
- 1 tablespoon toasted coconut

Directions

1. In a large bowl, mix all ingredients together; refrigerate, covered, overnight.

2. Divide porridge into serving bowls and top with peanut butter, and toasted coconut.

Nutritional Information per Serving:

Calories: 293; Total Fat: 27.5 g; Carbs: 10.7 g; Dietary Fiber: 4.3 g; Sugars: 5.6 g; Protein: 24.6 g; Cholesterol: 0 mg; Sodium: 35 mg

6. Spiced Salmon Frittata

Yield: 2 Servings

Total Time: 30 Minutes

Prep Time: 10 Minutes

Cook Time: 20 Minutes

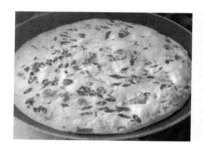

Ingredients:

- 1 tablespoon coconut oil
- 1 red onion, chopped
- 1 green pepper, chopped

- 2 garlic cloves, minced
- 1 ½ cups cherry tomatoes
- 1/2 teaspoon paprika
- 1 teaspoon cumin
- 1/2 cup wild-caught salmon
- 6 free-range eggs beaten
- Pinch of sea salt
- Pinch of pepper
- 2 tablespoons chopped cilantro

Directions:

1. Preheat oven to 350°F.

2. Melt butter in oven-safe skillet and sauté red onion and green pepper; stir in garlic and cook for about 2 minutes or until fragrant.

3. Stir in paprika, cumin, salt and pepper and cook for about 1 minute; stir in tomatoes and cook until soft.

4. Sprinkle with salmon and cover with eggs; season with salt and pepper and bake for about 15 minutes or until eggs are set.

5. Serve warm garnished with cilantro.

Nutritional Information per Serving:

Calories: 344; Total Fat: 22 g; Carbs: 16 g; Dietary Fiber: 4.2 g; Sugars: 8.4 g; Protein: 23.5 g; Cholesterol: 500 mg; Sodium: 325 mg

7. Spicy Mexican Breakfast Scramble

Yield: 2 Servings

Total Time: 20 Minutes

Prep Time: 10 Minutes

Cook Time: 10 Minutes

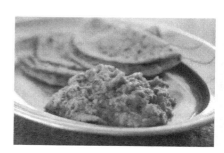

Ingredients

- 1 tablespoon coconut oil
- 1/4 red onion, diced
- 1/4 Bell Pepper, diced
- 1 tablespoon hot sauce
- 4 free-range eggs
- 1/2 teaspoon red pepper flakes, crushed
- 1/2 teaspoon cumin
- Pinch of sea salt
- Pinch of pepper
- 2 tablespoons freshly prepared salsa

Directions

1. Melt coconut oil in a nonstick skillet set over medium heat; stir in red onions and peppers and sauté for about 4 minutes or until onions are translucent.

2. Meanwhile, in a bowl, whisk together hot sauce, eggs, crushed red pepper flakes, cumin, salt and pepper until frothy;

3. add to onion mixture and cook, stirring, until eggs are set.

4. Season with salt and pepper and top with salsa. Serve immediately.

Nutrition Information per Serving:

Calories: 203; Total Fat: 15.9 g; Carbs: 4.7 g; Dietary Fiber: 1 g; Sugars: 2.7 g Protein: 11.8 g; Cholesterol: 327 mg; Sodium: 528 mg

8. Yummy Zucchini & Beef Frittata

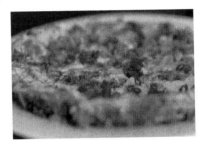

Yield: 4 Servings

Total Time: 35 Minutes

Prep Time: 15 Minutes

Cook Time: 20 Minutes

Ingredients:

- 1 tablespoon butter
- 1/2 red onion, minced
- 1 clove garlic, minced
- 8 ounce ground beef, crumbled
- 4 zucchini, thinly sliced
- 6 free-range eggs
- Pinch of sea salt
- Pinch of pepper

Directions:

1. Preheat oven to 350°F.

2. Sauté red onion in an oven-safe skillet with butter for about 3 minutes or until tender; add garlic, beef, and zucchini and cook for about 7 minutes or until zucchini is tender and beef is cooked through.

3. Season with salt and pepper and remove from heat; cover the zucchini mixture with egg and bake for about 10 minutes or until egg is set. Serve warm.

Nutritional Information per Serving:

Calories: 263; Total Fat: 13.3 g; Carbs: 8.6 g; Dietary Fiber: 2.5 g; Sugars: 4.5 g; Protein: 28.1 g; Cholesterol: 304 mg; Sodium: 229 mg

9. Detoxifying Rainbow Acai Bowl

Yield: 2 Servings

Total Time: 5 Minutes

Prep Time: 5 Minutes

Cook Time: N/A

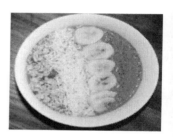

Ingredients
- 1/4 cup frozen raspberries
- 1/4 cup frozen blueberries
- 1/2 cup nonfat Greek yoghurt
- 1 teaspoon chia seeds
- 1 teaspoon acai powder
- 1 teaspoon vanilla protein powder

- 1 mango, sliced
- 1 small orange, segmented
- 1 tablespoon pistachios, chopped, toasted

Directions

1. In a blender, blend together, berries, yogurt, chia seed, acai powder, and mango until very smooth;
2. Spoon into two serving bowls and top each with fresh blueberries, strawberries, banana, orange and pistachios. Enjoy!

Nutrition info Per Serving:

Calories: 198; Total Fat: 2.9 g; Carbs: 11.5 g; Dietary Fiber: 6.4 g; Sugars: 6.6; Protein: 18.6 g; Cholesterol: 3 mg; Sodium: 31 mg

10. Choco Peanut Butter Milkshake

Yield: 1 Serving

Total Time: 5 Minutes

Prep Time: 5 Minutes

Cook Time: N/A

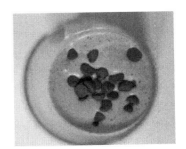

Ingredients

- 1 tablespoon natural peanut butter
- 1 tablespoon unsweetened cocoa powder
- 1 cup unsweetened coconut milk
- Pinch of sea salt

- 1 teaspoon liquid stevia
- 1 scoop protein powder

Directions

Blend all ingredients together until smooth. Enjoy!

Nutritional Information per Serving:

Calories: 664; Total Fat: 66 g; Carbs: 19.2 g; Dietary Fiber: 8.1 g; Sugars: 9.1 g; Protein: 31.6 g; Cholesterol: 0 mg; Sodium: 274 mg

11. Superfood Fruity Parfait

Yield: 2 Servings

Total Time: 10 Minutes

Prep Time: 10 Minutes

Cook Time: N/A

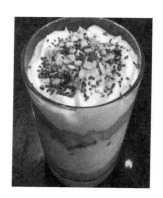

Ingredients

- 1 cup nonfat Greek yogurt
- 1 cup mixed berries
- 2 tablespoons crunchy whole-grain cereal
- 1 scoop vanilla protein powder
- 1 tablespoon flaxseed
- 1 tablespoon chia seeds

Directions

1. In a tall serving glass, alternate the layers of nonfat Greek yogurt, and mixed berries.

2. Top with crunchy whole grain cereal, flaxseed, chia seeds and protein powder.

Enjoy!

Nutritional Information per Serving:
Calories: 182; Total Fat: 3.8 g; Carbs: 17.3 g; Dietary Fiber: 4.7 g; Sugars: 14.5 g; Protein: 23.2 g; Cholesterol: 6 mg; Sodium: 53 mg

12. **Delicious Breakfast Turkey Casserole**

Yield: 6 Servings

Total Time: 50 Minutes

Prep Time: 5 Minutes

Cook Time: 45 Minutes

Ingredients
- 1 tablespoon coconut oil
- 1/2 pound ground turkey
- 1 large sweet potato, cut into slices
- 1/2 cup spinach
- 12 eggs
- Salt and pepper

Directions

1. Preheat oven to 350°F. Lightly coat a square baking tray with coconut oil and set aside.

2. In a skillet set over medium heat, brown ground turkey in coconut oil; season well and remove from heat.

3. Layer the potato slices onto the baking tray and top with raw spinach and ground turkey.

4. In a small bowl, whisk eggs, salt and pepper until well blended; pour over the mixture to cover completely; bake for about 45 minutes or until eggs are cooked through and the potatoes are tender.

5. Remove from oven and let cool a bit before serving.

Nutrition info Per Serving:
Calories: 247; Total Fat: 15.2 g; Carbs: 7 g; Dietary Fiber: 1.1 g; Sugars: 2.6; Protein: 22.1 g; Cholesterol: 366 mg; Sodium: 176 mg

13. Spicy Breakfast Scrambled Eggs

Yield: 2 Servings

Total Time: 30 Minutes

Prep Time: 10 Minutes

Cook Time: 20 Minutes

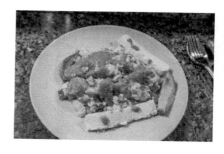

Ingredients

- 4 beaten eggs
- 1 tsp. extra virgin olive oil
- 1 small red onion, chopped
- 1 chopped red chilli

- 1 tsp. turmeric
- Splash of milk
- ½ cup diced tomatoes
- Parsley leaves, chopped
- Salt and pepper to taste

Directions

1.Sauté onion and chilli in extra virgin olive oil; stir in the eggs and milk; cook over medium-low heat until almost scrambled.

2.Stir in tomatoes, turmeric, and parsley. Season and serve in toast.

Nutritional Information Per Serving

Calories: 188; Total Fat: 11.6 g; Carbs: 8.6 g; Dietary fiber: 1.8 g; Sugars: 4.1 g; Protein: 12.9 g; Cholesterol: 329 mg; Sodium: 134 mg

14. Vegetable Breakfast Casserole

Yield: 6 Servings

Total Time: 1 Hour 30 Minutes

Prep Time: 30 Minutes

Cook Time: 60 Minutes

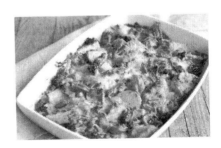

Ingredients

- 10 ounce bacon, chopped
- 1 cup diced red onion
- 1 cup shredded carrots

- ¾ cup diced bell pepper
- 2 cups chopped green beans
- 3 cups spinach
- 1 cup water
- 12 free-range eggs, beaten
- 1 teaspoon sea salt
- ½ teaspoon pepper

Directions

1. Preheat oven to 350°F. Coat a 9x13-inch casserole dish with olive oil cooking spray and set aside.

2. Cook bacon in a skillet over medium heat for about 10 minutes or until crispy; stir in red onions, carrots, bell pepper and green beans and continue cooking for about 5 minutes or until veggies are tender.

3. Stir in spinach and cook for 2 minutes or until wilted; remove from heat.

4. In a blender, blend together water, eggs and salt and well combined.

5. Transfer the vegetable mixture to the casserole and cover with egg mixture; stir well and bake for about 60 minutes or until eggs are set.

Nutritional Information per Serving:

Calories: 417; Total Fat: 28.5 g; Carbs: 9.4 g; Dietary Fiber: 2.7 g; Sugars: 3.7 g; Protein: 30.2 g; Cholesterol: 379 mg; Sodium: 1556 mg

15. Tasty Berry Omelet

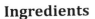

Yield: 1 Serving

Total Time: 17 Minutes

Prep Time: 10 Minutes

Cook Time: 7 Minutes

Ingredients

- 1 large egg
- 1 tablespoon almond milk
- ¼ teaspoon cinnamon
- ½ teaspoon rapeseed oil
- 100g cottage cheese
- 1 ½ cups chopped raspberries, blueberries, and strawberries

Directions

1. In a bowl, beat together the egg, milk and cinnamon until well blended.

2. Add oil to a nonstick pan set over medium heat. Add the egg mixture and swirl to cover the base evenly. Cook the egg mixture until set.

3. Transfer the omelet to a plate and sprinkle with cheese. Top with berries and roll up to serve.

Nutritional Information per Serving:

Calories: 298; Total Fat: 12.2 g; Carbs: 18.2 g; Dietary Fiber: 12 g; Protein: 22.5 g; Cholesterol: 149 mg; Sodium: 480 mg; Sugars: 9 g

16. Sausage & Broccoli Breakfast Quiche

Yield: 8 Servings

Total Time: 1 Hour 10 Minutes

Prep Time: 15 Minutes

Cook Time: 55 Minutes

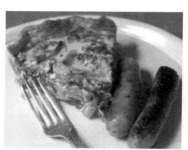

Ingredients

- 1 cup broccoli
- ½ pound breakfast sausage
- 2 cups almond flour
- 1 tablespoon sea salt
- 9 eggs
- 2 tablespoons coconut oil
- 2 tablespoons water

Directions

1. Steam the broccoli and set aside.Cook the sausage and set aside.

2. Blend almond flour and sea salt in a food processor until well combined.Add one egg and coconut oil and continue processing to form a ball.

3. Spread the dough on a quiche dish and top with broccoli and sausage.In a bowl, whisk the remaining eggs with water and pour over the broccoli and sausage.

4. Bake at 350°Ffor about 35 minutes or until firm and cooked through.

Nutritional Information per Serving:

Calories: 338; Total Fat: 23.8 g; Carbs: 6.2 g; Dietary Fiber: 3.3 g; Protein: 17.6 g; Cholesterol: 208 mg; Sodium: 520 mg; Sugars: 1.6 g

17. **Avocado Shrimp Omelet**

Yields: 2 Servings

Total Time: 40 Minutes

Prep Time: 10 Minutes

Cook Time: 30 Minutes

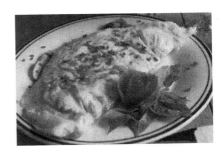

Ingredients

- 1/4 pound shrimp, peeled and de-veined
- 4 large free range eggs, beaten
- 1/2 medium avocado, diced
- 1 medium tomato, diced
- 1 tsp. coconut oil
- 1/8 tsp. freshly ground black pepper
- 1/4 tsp. sea salt
- 1 tbsp.   freshly chopped cilantro

Directions

1. Cook shrimp in a skillet set over medium heat until it turns pink; chop the cooked shrimp and set aside.In a small bowl, toss together avocado, tomato, and cilantro; season with sea salt and pepper and set aside,in a separate bowl, beat the eggs and set aside.

2. Set a skillet over medium heat; add coconut oil and heat until hot.

3. Add half of the egg to the skillet and tilt the skillet to cover the bottom. When almost cooked, add shrimp onto one side of the egg and fold in half. Cook for 1 minute more and top with the avocado-tomato mixture.Repeat with the remaining ingredients for the second omelet.

Nutritional Information Per Serving:

Calories: 344; Total Fat: 23.1 g; Carbs: 8.4 g; Dietary Fiber: 4.2 g; Protein: 27 g; Cholesterol: 491 mg; Sodium: 519 mg

18. **Yummy Breakfast Stir Fry**

Yield: 1 Serving

Total Time: 50 Minutes

Prep Time: 10 Minutes

Cook Time: 40 Minutes

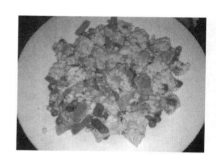

Ingredients

- 4 egg whites, beaten
- 2 small onions, chopped
- 1 green pepper, chopped
- 2 medium tomatoes, chopped
- A handful mushrooms, chopped
- ½ tablespoon extra-virgin olive oil,
- A pinch of sea salt
- Black olives, hot banana peppers and sliced cucumber, for serving

Directions

1. Add olive oil to a pan and add the green peppers.

2. Cover and cook on high heat for about 2 minutes then lower the heat and cook for 3 more minutes.

3. Next add the onions and the mushrooms and cover. Cook until tender then stir in the tomatoes. Sprinkle the salt, cover and simmer for about 15 minutes or until the melamen is soft and juicy.

4. Gently drizzle the egg whites over the melamen. Allow to cook without stirring for about a minute.

5. Roast the hot bananas peppers on your burner over medium heat, careful not burn them too much.

6. Serve the stir fry with whole wheat pita bread, black olives, roasted hot banana pepper and sliced cucumbers. You can also serve with traditional Mediterranean tea.

Enjoy!

Nutritional Information Per Serving:

Calories: 330; Total Fat: 9.3 g; Carbs: 17.4 g; Dietary Fiber: 13.1 g; Sugars: 3.7 g; Protein: 22.9 g; Cholesterol: 0 mg; Sodium: 209 mg

19. **Tasty Breakfast Wrap**

Yield: 1 Serving

Total Time: 50 Minutes

Prep Time: 10 Minutes

Cook Time: 40 Minutes

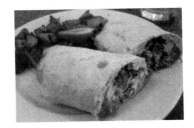

Ingredients

- 2 multi grain flax wraps
- 3 egg whites
- 1 ½ tbsp. extra virgin olive oil
- ¼ cup sun dried tomatoes
- ¼ cup fresh spinach, chopped
- ¼ cup crumbled feta cheese
- Sea salt and freshly ground pepper to taste

Directions

1. Heat the oil in a nonstick pan and sauté the tomatoes, spinach and egg whites until almost done then flip and cook the other side.

2. Add the crumbled feta to warm it up. Sprinkle with salt and pepper then remove from heat.

3. Heat the wraps on a dry pan then serve the egg mixture into the wraps and roll them up.

Enjoy!

Nutritional Information Per Serving:

Calories: 391; Total Fat: 33.1 g; Carbs: 17.4 g; Dietary Fiber: 1.8 g; Sugars: 2.3 g; Protein: 17.7 g; Cholesterol: 33 mg; Sodium: 529 mg

20. **Chocolate Pecan Smoothie**

Yield: 1 Serving

Total Time: 15 Minutes

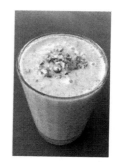

Prep Time: 10 Minutes

Cook Time: 5 Minutes

Ingredients:

- ¼ cup chopped pecans
- 2 tbsp. flaxseed meal
- 1/3 cup pasteurized egg whites
- 1 cup chocolate almond milk (unsweetened)
- 2 scoops low-carb vanilla protein
- Stevia, to taste
- 5 ice cubes

Directions

Combine all the ingredients in a blender and blend until very smooth. Enjoy!

Nutritional information Per Serving:

Calories: 390; Total Fat: 21 g; Total Carbs: 18 g; Dietary Fiber: 10 g; Protein: 39 g

The Lunch Recipes

21. Satisfying Turkey Lettuce Wraps

Yields: 4 Servings

Total Time: 35 Minutes

Prep Time: 15 Minutes

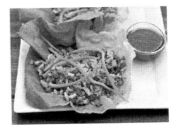

Cook Time: 20 Minutes

Ingredients

- 1/2 lb. ground turkey
- 1/2 small onion, finely chopped
- 1 garlic clove, minced
- 2 tablespoons extra virgin olive oil
- 1 head lettuce
- 1 teaspoon cumin
- 1/2 tablespoon fresh ginger, sliced
- 2 tablespoons apple cider vinegar
- 2 tablespoons freshly chopped cilantro
- 1 teaspoon freshly ground black pepper
- 1 teaspoon sea salt

Directions

1. Sauté garlic and onion in extra virgin olive oil until fragrant and translucent. Add turkey and cook well.

2. Stir in the remaining ingredients and continue cooking for 5 minutes more.

3. To serve, ladle a spoonful of turkey mixture onto a lettuce leaf and wrap. Enjoy!

Nutrition Information per Serving:

Calories: 192; Total Fat: 13.6 g; Carbs: 4.6 g; Dietary Fiber: 1 g; Sugars: 1.2 g Protein: 16.3 g; Cholesterol: 58 mg; Sodium: 535 mg

22. Grilled Steak Salad w/ Buttermilk-Avocado Buttermilk Dressing

Yield: 4 Servings

Total Time: 20 Minutes

Prep Time: 10 Minutes

Cook Time: 10 Minutes

Ingredients

For the salads

- Salad greens
- 2 plum tomatoes, sliced
- Leftover steak, sliced thinly

Dressing

- 2/3 cup buttermilk
- half of an avocado
- 8-10 chives
- 1 clove of garlic, chopped
- 4 fresh basil leaves
- 1 teaspoon dried minced red onion
- A sprig fresh rosemary
- 1/2 teaspoon dried dill
- A few leaves of fresh parsley
- 1/2 liquid stevia
- pinch of chicory powder
- 1/4 teaspoon sea salt
- Pinch of pepper

Directions

1. Mix salad ingredients and divide among serving plates; top each with steak slices, tomato, and mango.

2. In a food processor or blend, blend together dressing ingredients until very smooth; pour over salad and toss to coat well. Enjoy!

Nutritional Information per Serving:

Calories: 34; Total Fat: 11.2 g; Carbs: 17 g; Dietary Fiber: 4.5 g; Sugars: 16.1 g; Protein: 38.8 g; Cholesterol: 1.3 mg; Sodium: 311 mg

23. Lentil Coconut Curry Soup

Yield: 4 Servings

Total Time: 45 Minutes

Prep Time: 5 Minutes

Cook Time: 40 Minutes

Ingredients

- 1 tbsp. coconut oil
- 2 cloves garlic, minced
- 1 large onion, chopped
- 1 tbsp. minced ginger
- ½ tsp. hot red pepper flakes
- 2 tbsp. tomato paste
- 2 tbsp. curry powder
- 1.5 cups dry red lentils

- 1 400g can diced tomatoes
- 1 400ml can coconut milk
- 4 cups vegetable broth
- 1 cup chopped spinach or kale
- A pinch of Sea salt and pepper
- Garnish: vegan sour cream and chopped cilantro

Directions

1. Heat coconut oil in a stockpot set over medium heat;

2. stir in garlic, onion, and ginger and sauté for about 4 minutes or until fragrant and onion is translucent.

3. Stir in tomato paste, red pepper flakes, and curry powder; cook for 1 minute more and stir in lentils, diced tomatoes, coconut milk and vegetable broth.

4. Cook, covered for about 30 minutes or until lentils are tender; season with salt and pepper.

5. To serve, stir in spinach or kale and garnish with vegan sour cream and cilantro. Enjoys

Nutritional Information per Serving:

Calories: 220; Total Fat: 13.3 g; Carbs: 15.8 g; Dietary Fiber: 1.5 g; Sugars: 2.9 g; Protein: 20.7 g; Cholesterol: 65 mg; Sodium: 1272 mg

24. Steamed Salmon w/ Fennel & Fresh Herbs

Yield: 4 Servings

Total Time: 21 Minutes

Prep Time: 15 Minutes

Cook Time: 6 Minutes

Ingredients

- 1 tablespoon extra-virgin olive oil
- 6 ounces wild salmon fillets, skinless
- Fennel fronds
- 1 tablespoon chopped parsley
- 1 tablespoon chopped dill
- 1 tablespoon chopped chives
- 1 tablespoon chopped tarragon
- 1 tablespoon chopped basil
- 1 tablespoon chopped shallot
- 1 tablespoon lemon juice

Directions

1. Lightly oil a steamer basket with olive oil; add salmon and fennel wedges and steam for about 6 minutes.

2. In a bowl, combine the chopped herbs, extra virgin olive oil, and shallot and lemon juice; stir until well combined.

3. Season and spoon over cooked fish.

Nutritional Information per Serving:

Calories: 98; Total Fat: 6.3 g; Carbs: 2.5 g; Dietary Fiber: 0.9 g; sugars: trace; Protein: 8.9 g; Cholesterol: 19 mg; Sodium: 33 mg

25. Fried Tofu w/ Spring Greens

Yields: 3 Servings

Total Time: 35 Minutes

Prep Time: 10 Minutes

Cook Time: 25 Minutes

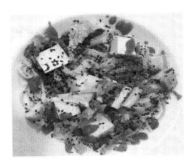

Ingredients

- 2 tablespoons extra virgin olive oil
- 14- ounce extra-firm tofu, sliced
- 1 medium onion, thinly sliced
- 1 medium yellow or red bell pepper, chopped
- 2 teaspoons grated fresh ginger
- 12 ounces spring greens, chopped
- 3 tablespoons teriyaki sauce
- 1/4 cup toasted cashews, chopped

Directions

1. Add half oil to a pan set over medium heat. Add tofu and fry until golden. Transfer to a plate.

2. Add the remaining oil to the pan and sauté onion until translucent.

3. Stir in bell pepper and continue sautéing until onion is tender and golden. Stir in ginger and greens until wilted.

4. Stir in tofu and season with teriyaki sauce. Top with toasted cashews to serve.

Nutritional Information per Serving:

Calories: 338; Total Fat: 22.7 g; Carbs: 17.8 g; Dietary Fiber: 6.9 g; Protein: 19.3 g; Cholesterol: 0 mg; Sodium: 962 mg; sugars: 7.6 g

26. Cashews-and Pretzel-Crusted Tofu

Yield: 4 Servings

Total Time: 35 Minutes

Prep Time: 15 Minutes

Cook Time: 20 Minutes

Ingredients

- 1 cup whole wheat flour
- 1 package (16-ounce) extra firm tofu, chopped into 8 slices
- ¾ cup raw cashews
- 2 cups pretzel sticks
- 1 tbsp. extra virgin olive oil
- 1 cup unsweetened almond milk
- 2 tsp. chili powder
- 2 tsp. garlic powder
- 2 tsp. onion powder
- 1 tsp. lemon pepper
- ¼ tsp. black pepper
- ½ tsp. sea salt

Directions

1. Preheat your oven to 400°F.Line a baking sheet with baking paper and set aside.

2. In a food processor, pulse together cashews and pretzel sticks until coarsely ground.

3. Combine garlic, onion, chili powder, lemon pepper, and salt in a small bowl.

4. In a large bowl, combine half of the spice mixture and flour.

Preheat oven to 400F. Line a large baking sheet with parchment paper

5. Combine pretzel sticks and cashews in a food processor and pulse a few times, until coarsely ground. Add almond milk to a separate bowl.

6. In another bowl, combine cashew mixture, salt, pepper and olive oil; mix well.

7. Sprinkle tofu slices with the remaining half of the spice mixture and coat each with the flour and then dip in almond mil; coat with the cashew mixture and bake for about 18 minutes or until golden brown.

8. Serve the baked tofu with favorite vegan salad.

Nutritional Information per Serving:

Calories: 451; Total Fat: 19 g; Carbs: 19.2 g; Dietary Fiber: 3.9 g; Sugars: 3.3 g; Protein: 13.7 g; Cholesterol: 0 mg; Sodium: 709 mg

27. Teriyaki Fish w/ Zucchini

Yields: 2 Servings

Total Time: 20 Minutes

Prep Time: 10 Minutes

Cook Time: 10 Minutes

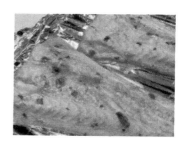

Ingredients

- 2 (6-ounce) salmon fillets
- 7 tablespoons teriyaki sauce (low-sodium)
- 2 tablespoons sesame seeds
- 2 teaspoons canola oil
- 4 scallions, chopped
- 2 small zucchini, thinly sliced

Directions

1. Mix fish with 5 tablespoons of teriyaki sauce in a zip-top bag and marinate for at least 20 minutes.

2. In a skillet set over medium heat, toast sesame seeds; set aside. Drain the marinated fish and discard the marinade.

3. Add fish to the skillet and cook for about 5 minutes; remove fish from skillet and keep warm.

4. Add oil, scallions and zucchini to the skillet and sauté for about 4 minutes or until browned.

5. Stir in the remaining teriyaki sauce and sprinkle with toasted sesame seeds; serve with fish.

Nutritional Information per Serving:

Calories: 408; Total Fat: 19.9 g; Carbs: 18.1 g; Dietary Fiber: 4.3 g; Protein: 40.3 g; Cholesterol: 75 mg; Sodium: 2505 mg; sugars: 11.7 g

28. Italian Fish Stew

Yields: 2 Servings

Total Time: 40 Minutes

Prep Time: 15 Minutes

Cook Time: 25 Minutes

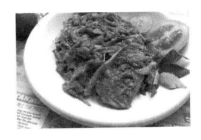

Ingredients

- 4 200g Kingklip fish fillets
- 2 onions, finely chopped
- 4 garlic cloves, minced
- 2 tins peeled, chopped tomato
- 4 tbsp. tomato paste
- 250ml white wine
- ½ tsp. parsley, chopped
- ¼ tsp. dried oregano
- salt and pepper to taste
- ½ cup olive oil
- 1 cup water

Directions

6. Preheat oven to 360C. Sauté onion and garlic on a pot then add tinned tomatoes and tomato paste and stir.

7. Pour the wine, parsley, oregano, salt, pepper, and water. Stir well and bring to a simmer.

8. Let it simmer for 10-15 minutes to reduce and thicken.

9. Meanwhile, place your fish in baking dish.

10. When sauce is nice and thick, pour it over fish and sprinkle with a little extra oregano.

11. Cover the dish with foil and place in the oven to cook for 20 minutes.

12. Take foil off and return to oven uncovered and cook for another 10 minutes.

13. Tip: If the sauce is a little runny when fish comes out, place sauce in another pot and put on heat to reduce a little more. Then pour back over fish.

Nutritional Information per Serving:

Calories: 315; Total Fat: 8 g; Carbs: 12 g; Dietary Fiber: 1.5 g; Sugars: 2.9 g; Protein: 37 g; Cholesterol: 54 mg; Sodium: 1302 mg

29. Grilled Tuna w/ Bean & Tomato Salad

Yields: 4 Servings

Total Time: 19 Minutes

Prep Time: 15 Minutes

Cook Time: 4 Minutes

Ingredients

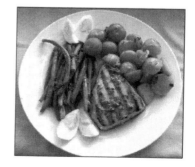

- 1 1/2 tablespoons extra-virgin olive oil
- 3 scallions, thinly sliced
- 1 tablespoon fresh lemon juice
- 1/4 cup fresh tarragon leaves
- 1 (15 ounces) can beans, drained, rinsed
- 1 pound heirloom tomatoes, cored, diced
- Sea salt
- 4 (8 ounce) tuna steaks

Directions

1. In a bowl, mix together oil, scallions, lemon juice, tarragon, beans, tomatoes, and salt; set aside.

2. Lightly grease the grill grates with oil and heat to medium. Season tuna with salt and grill for about 4 minutes or until cooked through. Serve tuna with bean salad.

Nutritional Information per Serving:

Calories: 505; Total Fat: 19.8g; Carbs: 9.4g; Dietary Fiber: 4g; Protein: 70.4g; Cholesterol: 111mg; Sodium: 123mg; sugars: 1.8g

30. Steamed Bass with Fennel, Parsley, and Capers

Yields: 2 Servings

Total Time: 30 Minutes

Prep Time: 15 Minutes

Cook Time: 15 Minutes

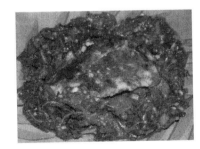

Ingredients

- 2 5-ounce portions of striped bass

- 2 tablespoons extra-virgin olive oil
- 1/2 lemon, juiced
- 1 fennel bulb, sliced
- 1/4 medium onion, sliced
- 1/4 cup chopped parsley
- 1 tablespoon capers, rinsed
- 1/2 teaspoon sea salt
- Chopped parsley and olive oil, for garnish

Directions

1. Add lemon juice, fennel and onion to a pan and cover with 1-inch water; bring the mixture to a gentle boil. Lower heat and simmer for about 5 minutes.

2. Add seasoned fish and sprinkle with parsley and capers; cover and simmer for about 10 minutes.

3. Transfer to a serving bowl and drizzle with extra virgin olive oil and top with more parsley to serve.

Nutritional Information per Serving:

Calories: 325; Total Fat: 24.6g; Carbs: 10.54g; Dietary Fiber: 4.3g; Protein: 10.9g; Cholesterol: 0mg; Sodium: 661mg; sugars: 0.7g

31. Turkey & Coconut Soup

Yield: 2 Servings

Total Time: 40 Minutes

Prep Time: 10 Minutes

Cook Time: 30 Minutes

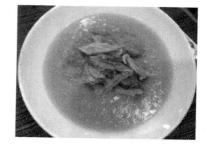

Ingredients

- 1 tsp. coconut oil
- 1 red onion, finely sliced
- 1 ginger, finely chopped
- 1 clove garlic, finely chopped
- 1 lemon grass, bashed with a rolling pin
- 2 sticks celery, diced
- 1/4 cup coconut milk
- ½ cup vegetable stock
- 8 oz. turkey, cooked, roughly chopped
- 1/8 tsp. sea salt
- 1/8 tsp. black pepper
- 1 cup coriander, finely chopped
- 1 cup spinach, roughly chopped
- 2 tbsp. fresh lime juice

Directions

1. Add coconut oil to a medium pan set over medium heat; stir in red onions and sauté for about 5 minutes or until translucent.

2. Add ginger and garlic and sauté for about 3 minutes or until garlic is golden.

3. Stir in lemon grass, celery, coconut milk, and vegetable sock; bring to a simmer. Simmer for about 15 minutes or until celery is soft.

4. Stir in turkey, salt and black pepper; cook for about 5 minutes or until turkey is cooked heated through.

5. Remove from heat and stir in coriander and spinach; serve into soup bowls and sprinkle with a squeeze of lime juice and coriander.

Nutritional Information per Serving:

Calories: 327; Total Fat: 15.4 g; Carbs: 11.2 g; Dietary Fiber: 3.4 g; Sugars: 4.4 g; Protein: 35.8 g; Cholesterol: 86 mg; Sodium: 276 mg

32. Crunchy Kale & Almond Salad with Roasted Chicken

Yield: 6 Servings

Total Time: 55 Minutes

Prep Time: 10 Minutes

Cook Time: 45 Minutes

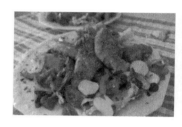

Ingredients:

Salad

- 2 tablespoons extra virgin olive oil
- 1 pound Lacinato kale, sliced into thin strips
- 1/2 cup roasted almonds
- Pinch of sea salt
- Pinch of pepper

Roasted Chicken

- 2 pounds chicken thighs
- Pinch of sea salt
- Pinch of pepper
- 2 tablespoons apple cider vinegar
- 1 tablespoon extra-virgin olive oil
- 1/4 cup rosemary

- 1/4 cup sage

Directions:

1. Place kale in a bowl and add olive oil; massage olive oil with hands into kale until kale is tender; sprinkle with salt and pepper and toss with toasted almonds.

2. Preheat oven to 375°F. Sprinkle chicken with salt and pepper and place in a baking; add vinegar and olive oil and season with rosemary and sage.

3. Roast for about 45 minutes or until chicken is cooked through. Serve chicken with kale and almond salad.

Nutritional Information per Serving:

Calories: 454; Total Fat: 22.8 g; Carbs: 15.6 g; Dietary Fiber: 4.8 g; Sugars: 1.3 g; Protein: 48.4 g; Cholesterol: 135 mg; Sodium: 243 mg

33. Chicken w/Red Onions & Kale (Served with Chili-Tomato Salsa)

Yield: 1 Serving

Total Time: 40 Minutes

Prep Time: 20 Minutes

Cook Time: 20 Minutes

Ingredients:

- Juice of 1/4 lemon
- 2 teaspoons ground turmeric

- 1 tablespoon extra-virgin olive oil
- 4 ounces chicken breast, skinless, boneless
- ¼ cup chopped kale
- 1 teaspoon chopped ginger
- 1 large red onion, sliced
- ¼ cup buckwheat

For the salsa

- 1 large tomato, finely chopped
- 1 tablespoon capers, finely chopped
- 1 bird's eye chili, finely chopped
- Juice of 1/4 lemon
- ½ cup parsley, finely chopped

Directions

1. Make salsa: mix chopped tomato, capers, chili, lemon juice, and parsley in a large bowl.

2. Preheat your oven to 450°F.

3. In a large bowl, mix lemon juice, 1 teaspoon turmeric, and a splash of extra virgin olive oil; add the chicken and stir to combine well. Marinate for about 10 minutes.

4. Set an ovenproof pan over medium heat and add the chicken; cook for about 4 minutes per side or until lightly browned.

5. Transfer to the preheated oven and bake for about 10 minutes remove from the oven and remove the chicken from oven and keep warm.

6. In the meantime, steam kale in a steamer for about 5 minutes.

7. Fry ginger and red onion in a splash of extra virgin olive oil until tender; stir in kale and cook for about 1 minute.

8. Follow package instructions to cook buckwheat with the remaining turmeric.

9. Serve the buckwheat with chicken, veggies and salsa.

Nutritional Information per Serving:

Calories: 335; Total Fat: 11.6g; Carbs: 2.6g; Dietary Fiber: 4.3g; Protein: 22.5g; Cholesterol: 51mg; Sodium: 224mg; sugars: 5.8g

34. Tasty Chicken Greek Salad

Yield: 4 Servings

Total Time: 25 Minutes

Prep Time: 10 Minutes

Cook Time: 15 Minutes

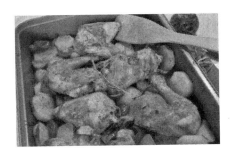

Ingredients

- 330g cooked chicken, cubed
- ½ cup black olives, sliced
- ½ cup red onion, chopped
- 1/3 cup red wine vinegar
- 6 cups romaine lettuce, roughly torn
- 2 tomatoes, diced
- 2 tbsp. extra virgin olive oil
- 1 cucumber, peeled and chopped
- ½ cup crumbled feta cheese
- 1 tbsp. fresh dill, chopped or 1 tsp dried oregano

- ¼ tsp freshly ground pepper
- 1 tsp garlic powder
- Kosher salt of flaky sea salt to taste

Directions

1. Whisk olive oil, red wine vinegar, dill/ oregano, salt, garlic powder and pepper in a large salad bowl.

2. Toss in the cubed chicken, lettuce, tomatoes, olives, cucumber, onion and feta cheese and mix well until evenly coated.

3. Note: if you don't have ready chicken, poach 450g chicken breast in a medium saucepan with salted water for about 15 minutes until cooked through.

4. Set aside to cool then cut it in cubes.

Nutritional Information per Serving:

Calories: 300; Total Fat: 15.7 g; Carbs: 11.5 g; Dietary Fiber: 2.6 g; Sugars: 5.3 g; Protein: 28.4 g; Cholesterol: 80 mg; Sodium: 419 mg; sugars: 5.8g

35. Spiced Turkey Served with Avocado Relish

Yield: 2 Servings

Total Time: 15Minutes

Prep Time: 10 Minutes

Cook Time: 5 Minutes

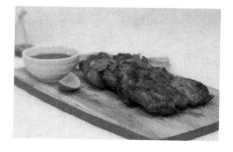

Ingredients

- 225g turkey cutlets
- ½ tsp 5-spice powder
- 2 tbsp. extra virgin olive oil
- 1 tbsp. chili powder
- A good pinch kosher salt

For the avocado relish:

- ½ avocado, diced1 seedless grapefruit, cut into segments and discarding the membranes
- 1 small Vidalia onion, minced
- 1 tsp. red wine vinegar
- 1 tbsp. fresh cilantro, chopped
- 1 tsp natural honey

Directions

1. Combine the avocado, grapefruit segments, onion, honey, vinegar and cilantro and toss well to combine.

2. Next, combine all the spices for the turkey in a shallow bowl then dredge the cutlets in the spice mix.

3. Add the oil to a pan over medium heat and sear the turkey until cooked to desired doneness for about 3-5 minutes on each side.

4. Serve hot with the relish.Enjoy!

Nutritional Information per Serving:

Calories: 440; Total Fat: 30.1 g; Carbs: 9.7 g; Dietary Fiber: 5.4 g; Sugars: 2 g; Protein: 34.8 g; Cholesterol: 85 mg; Sodium: 121 mg

36. Yummy Seafood Salad

Yield: 4 Servings

Total Time: 15 Minutes

Prep Time: 10 Minutes

Cook Time: 5 Minutes

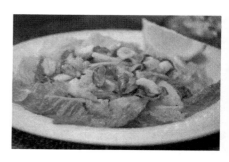

Ingredients

- 300g lump crab meat
- 4 medium-dry scallops, cut into quarters with the tough muscle removed
- 6 cherry tomatoes, cut in half
- 3 tbsp. white wine vinegar
- 1 small ruby red grapefruit, peeled and cut into segments with the membranes and seeds removed
- 1 avocado, diced
- 1 tsp Dijon mustard
- 2 tbsp. extra virgin olive oil
- 1 shallot, minced
- 3 cups romaine lettuce, shredded
- ¼ tsp freshly ground pepper
- Flaky sea salt to taste

Directions

1. Add some water to a small saucepan and bring to a boil then add in the scallops and cook until opaque and firm for about a minute. Drain then rinse under cold water.

2. Whisk the mustard, shallot, salt, pepper and vinegar in a medium bowl then slowly whisk in the olive oil.

3. Toss in the scallops and the crab in the dressing and toss well until evenly coated.

4. Combine the avocado, tomatoes, lettuce and the grapefruit then add the scallop mixture into the tomato mixture and toss well to combine.

Enjoy!

Nutritional Information per Serving:

Calories: 286; Total Fat: 23.6 g; Carbs: 14.9 g; Dietary Fiber: 5.9 g; Sugars: 5.6 g; Protein: 18.7 g; Cholesterol: 52 mg; Sodium: 501 mg

37. Chicken with Greek Salad

Yield: 4 Servings

Total Time: 35 Minutes

Prep Time: 15 Minutes

Cook Time: 20 Minutes

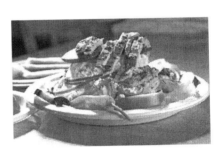

Ingredients

- 2 1/2 cups chopped chicken(cooked)
- 2 tbsp. extra-virgin olive oil
- 6 cups chopped romaine lettuce
- 1/4 tsp. freshly ground pepper
- 1 tbsp. chopped fresh dill
- 1/2 cup sliced ripe black olives
- 1/2 cup finely chopped red onion
- 1 cucumber, peeled, seeded and chopped
- 2 medium tomatoes, chopped

- 1/3 cup red-wine vinegar
- 1/2 cup crumbled feta cheese
- 1 tsp.   garlic powder
- 1/4 tsp. sea salt

Directions

1. In a large bowl, whisk together extra virgin olive oil, vinegar, garlic powder, dill, sea salt and pepper.

2. Add chicken, lettuce, cucumber, tomatoes, feta, and olives and toss to combine well. Enjoy!

Nutritional Information Per Serving:

Calories: 305; Total Fat: 15.8 g; Carbs: 11.8 g; Dietary Fiber: 2.7 g; Sugars: 5.3 g; Protein: 30 g; Cholesterol: 84 mg; Sodium: 539 mg

38. Chicken w/ Spicy Cauliflower Couscous

Yield: 4 Servings

Total Time: 35 Minutes

Prep Time: 15 Minutes

Cook Time: 20 Minutes

Ingredients

- 2 tbsp. extra virgin olive oil
- 1 cup roughly chopped cauliflower
- 1 tbsp. capers
- tsp. ground turmeric

- 1 tbsp. fresh lemon juice
- 1 chilli, finely chopped
- ¼ cup finely chopped red onions
- ¼ cup sun dried tomatoes
- 1 chicken breast (100g)
- 1 tsp. finely chopped fresh ginger
- ¼ cup finely diced carrots
- 1 clove garlic, finely diced
- 1 tbsp. chopped parsley

Directions

1. Roughly chop the cauliflower and set aside.

2. Heat a tablespoon of extra virgin olive oil in a pan set over medium high heat; stir in garlic, ginger, and chilli and sauté until tender.

3. Stir in cauliflower, carrots and turmeric and cook for about 5 minutes; remove the pan from heat and transfer the content to a large bowl. Add tomatoes and parsley; mix well. Set aside.

4. Cook chicken in the remaining oil over medium heat for about 6 minutes per side or until cooked through; stir in capers, lemon juice, and a tablespoon of water.

5. Combine cauliflower couscous with the chicken sauce and serve.

Enjoy!

Nutritional Information Per Serving:

Calories: 166; Total Fat: 9.8 g; Carbs: 5.8 g; Dietary Fiber: 1.8 g; Sugars: 1.4 g; Protein: 15.1 g; Cholesterol: 37 mg; Sodium: 146 mg

39. Salmon w/ celery Salad, Rocket & Caramelized Chicory

Yield: 1 Serving

Total Time: 25 Minutes

Prep Time: 15 Minutes

Cook Time: 10 Minutes

Ingredients

- 100g skinless salmon fillet
- 1 tsp. extra virgin olive oil
- 20g red onion, thinly sliced
- 1 tbsp. capers
- Juice of ¼ lemon
- 10g parsley
- 5g celery leaves
- 50g rocket
- 100g cherry tomatoes, halved
- ¼ avocado, peeled, stoned and diced
- 1 head (70g) chicory, halved lengthways
- 2 tsp. brown sugar

Directions

1. Preheat your oven to 450°F.

2. Make the dressing: in a food processor, combine capers, lemon juice, parsley, and 2 teaspoons of extra virgin olive oil; process until smooth.

3. Make the salad: in a salad bowl, combine avocado, red onion, celery, tomatoes, and rocket; set aside.

4. Rub fish with oil and sear in a hot frying pan for about 1 minute or until caramelized; transfer to a baking tray and roast in the oven for about 6 minutes.

5. In a small bowl, mix the remaining oil with brown sugar and brush over the cut sides of chicory; arrange chicory, cut side down, on a hot frying pan and cook for about for about 3 minutes or until caramelized and tender.

6. To serve, toss the salad in the lemon dressing and serve with caramelized chicory and salmon. Enjoy!

Nutritional Information Per Serving:

Calories: 342; Total Fat: 21.4 g; Carbs: 19 g; Dietary Fiber: 6.5 g; Sugars: 10.8 g; Protein: 23.3 g; Cholesterol: 44 mg; Sodium: 332 mg

40. Grilled Sardines w/ Wilted Arugula

Yield: 4 Servings

Total Time: 25 Minutes

Prep Time: 15 Minutes

Cook Time: 10 Minutes

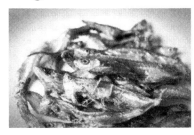

Ingredients

- 2 tsp. extra-virgin olive oil
- 16 fresh sardines, innards and gills removed
- 2 large bunches baby arugula, trimmed
- Sea salt
- Freshly ground black pepper
- Lemon wedges, for garnish

Directions

1. Prepare your outdoor grill or a stove-top griddle.

2. Rinse arugula under running water; shake off excess water and arrange them on a platter; set aside.

3. Rinse sardines in water and rub to remove scales; wipe them dry and combine with extra virgin olive oil in a large bowl.

4. Toss to coat. Place the sardines over the grill and grill for about 3 minutes per side or until golden brown and crispy.

5. Season with sea salt and pepper and immediately transfer to the platter lined with arugula. Serve right away garnished with lemon wedges.

Enjoy!

Nutritional Information Per Serving:

Calories: 222; Total Fat: 13.4 g; Carbs: 0.4 g; Dietary Fiber: trace; Sugars: trace; Protein: 23.9 g; Cholesterol: 136 mg; Sodium: 488 mg

41. Healthy Salmon Super Salad

Yield: 2 Serving

Total Time: 10 Minutes

Prep Time: 10 Minutes

Cook Time: N/A

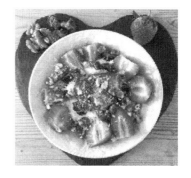

Ingredients

- 20 g red onion, sliced
- 1 tsp. extra virgin olive oil
- 1 large Medjool date, chopped
- 1 tbsp. capers
- ¼ cup rocket
- 1/2 avocado, peeled, stoned and sliced
- 100 g smoked salmon slices
- ¼ cup chicory leaves
- 2 tbsp. chopped walnuts
- 1 tbsp. fresh lemon juice
- ¼ cup chopped parsley
- ¼ cup chopped celery leaves

Directions

Arrange salad leaves in a large bowl or a plate; mix the remaining ingredients well and serve over the salad leaves.

Nutritional Information Per Serving:

Calories: 261; Total Fat: 20 g; Carbs: 10.4 g; Dietary Fiber: 5.1 g; Sugars: 3.8 g; Protein: 23.3 g; Cholesterol: 22 mg; Sodium: 178 mg

42. Fish w/ Olives, Tomatoes & Capers

Yield: 4 Servings

Total Time: 25 Minutes

Prep Time: 10 Minutes

Cook Time: 15 Minutes

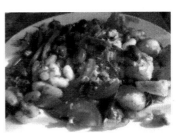

Ingredients

- 4 tsp. extra virgin olive oil, divided
- 2 cups fresh baby spinach leaves
- 4 (5-ounce) sea bass fillets
- 2 tbsp. capers
- 1/2 cup pitted black olives, chopped
- 1 cup canned diced tomatoes, with juice
- 1/2 cup white wine
- 1 small onion, diced
- 1/4 tsp. crushed red pepper
- Sea salt and pepper

Directions

1. Heat 2 teaspoons of extra virgin olive oil in a large nonstick skillet set over medium high heat.

2. Add fish and cook for about 3 minutes per side or until opaque in the center.

3. Transfer the cooked fish to a plate and keep warm.

4. Add the remaining oil to the skillet and sauté onion for about 2 minutes or until translucent.

5. Stir in wine and cook for about 2 minutes or until liquid is reduced by half.

6. Stir in capers, tomatoes, olives, and red pepper and cook for about 3 minutes more. Add spinach and cook, stirring for about 3 minutes or until silted. Stir in sea salt and pepper and spoon sauce over fish. Serve immediately.

Nutritional Information Per Serving:

Calories: 279; Total Fat: 10.4 g; Carbs: 6 g; Dietary Fiber: 2 g; Sugars: 2.2 g; Protein: 34.8 g; Cholesterol: 75 mg; Sodium: 414 mg

43. **Healthy Chicken Curry**

Yield: 1 Serving

Total Time: 30 Minutes

Prep Time: 10 Minutes

Cook Time: 20 Minutes

Ingredients

- 100 grams chicken, diced
- ¼ cup chicken broth
- Pinch of turmeric
- Dash of onion powder
- 1 tablespoon minced red onion
- Pinch of garlic powder
- ¼ teaspoon curry powder
- Pinch of sea salt
- Pinch of pepper
- Stevia

- Pinch of cayenne

Directions

In a small saucepan, stir spices in chicken broth until dissolved; stir in chicken, garlic, onion, and stevia and cook until chicken is cooked through and liquid is reduced by half. Serve hot.

Nutritional Information per Serving:

Calories: 170; Total Fat: 3.5 g; Carbs: 2.3 g; Dietary Fiber: 0.6 g; Sugars: 0.8 g; Protein: 30.5 g; Cholesterol: 77 mg; Sodium: 255 mg

44. Healthy Chicken Super Salad

Yield: 2 Serving

Total Time: 20 Minutes

Prep Time: 10 Minutes

Cook Time: 10 Minutes

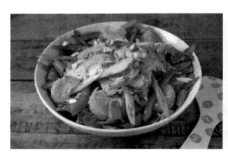

Ingredients

- 1 red onion, sliced
- 1 tsp. extra virgin olive oil
- 1 large date, chopped
- 1 tbsp. capers
- ¼ cup rocket
- ½ avocado, peeled, stoned and sliced
- 100 g chicken slices
- ¼ cup chicory leaves

- 2 tbsp. chopped walnuts
- 1 tbsp. fresh lemon juice
- ¼ cup chopped parsley
- ¼ cup chopped celery leaves

Directions

Arrange salad leaves in a large bowl or a plate; mix the remaining ingredients well and serve over the salad leaves.

Nutritional Information Per Serving:

Calories: 288; Total Fat: 18.5 g; Carbs: 14.7 g; Dietary Fiber: 6.1 g; Sugars: 5.8 g; Protein: 18.6 g; Cholesterol: 39 mg; Sodium: 181 mg

45. Salmon Salad in Avocado Cups

Yield: 2 Serving

Total Time: 30 Minutes

Prep Time: 10 Minutes

Cook Time: 20 Minutes

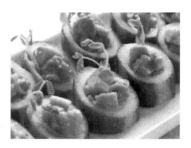

Ingredients

- 1 medium-sized salmon fillet
- 1 pc. shallot, diced
- ¼ cup mayo
- ½ juice of lime
- 2 tsps. fresh dill, chopped
- 1 tbsp. ghee
- 1 large avocado, sliced in half and pitted

- salt and pepper to taste

Directions

1. Preheat oven at 400F

2. Place the salmon fillet on a baking sheet and drizzle it with ghee and juice of lime.

3. Season with salt and pepper and place in the oven to cook for 20-25 minutes.

4. When done, allow the salmon to cook for a few minutes and shred using a fork.

5. Place the salmon in a bowl, add the diced shallot, and mix well.

6. Add the dill and mayo to the salmon mixture and combine well. Set aside.

7. Remove the insides of the avocado halves making sure that the skin is still intact to make cups.

8. Mash the avocado meat in a bowl and then add to the salmon mixture. Combine well.

9. Transfer the avocado and tuna salad back to the avocado cups and serve.

Nutritional Information per Serving:

Calories: 463; Total Fat: 35 g; Carbs: 6.4 g; Dietary Fiber: 1.5 g; Sugars: 2.9 g; Protein: 27 g; Cholesterol: 613 mg; Sodium: 1472 mg

46. Beef Shred Salad

Yield: 4 Servings

Total Time: 20 Minutes

Prep Time: 10 Minutes

Cook Time: 10 Minutes

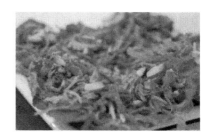

Ingredients

- 2 cups beef, shredded
- 1 yellow pepper, sliced thin lengthwise
- 1 white onion, sliced lengthwise
- 6 pcs. butter lettuce
- 2 tsp. mayo
- 1/8 tsp. chili flakes

Directions

1. Place the butter lettuces on a serving plate. Spread mayo on the lettuce and top with the shredded beef.

2. Place pepper slices and onions on top and season with chili flakes.

3. Serve as it is or rolled.

Nutritional Information per Serving:

Calories: 338; Total Fat: 25 g; Carbs: 2.4 g; Dietary Fiber: 1.7 g; Sugars: 0.3 g; Protein: 24 g; Cholesterol: 214 mg; Sodium: 1209 mg

47. Delicious Baked Tilapia in Garlic & Olive Oil

Yields: 4 Servings

Total Time: 35 Minutes

Prep Time: 15 Minutes

Cook Time: 30 Minutes

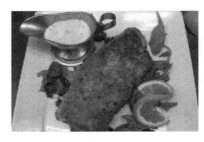

Ingredients

- 4 (4 ounce) tilapia fillets
- 4 cloves crushed garlic
- 3 tablespoon extra-virgin olive oil
- 1 chopped onion
- 1/4 teaspoon salt

Directions

1. Rub the tilapia fillets with garlic and arrange them in a baking dish.

2. Drizzle the fish with olive oil until well coated and top with onion.

3. Refrigerate the fish, covered, for at least 8 hours or overnight to soak in the marinade.

4. When ready, preheat your oven to 350°F (175°C).

5. Transfer the fish fillets to a 9x13 inch baking dish; pour over the marinade mixture and sprinkle with salt. Bake the fish for about 30 minutes.

Nutritional Information per Serving:

Calories: 194; Total Fat: 11.6g; Carbs: 2.6g; Dietary Fiber: 0.6g; Protein: 21.4g; Cholesterol: 0mg; Sodium: 154mg; sugars: 1.2g

48. Tilapia with Herbs

Yield: 1 Serving

Total Time: 25 Minutes

Prep Time: 10 Minutes

Cook Time: 15 Minutes

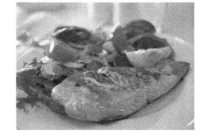

Ingredients
- 100 grams of Tilapia fish
- 1 tablespoon chopped red onion
- 1 clove garlic, minced
- 2 tablespoons fresh lemon juice
- Fresh parsley
- Pinch of dill
- Pinch of salt & pepper

Directions:
1. Sauté fish in a splash of fresh lemon juice and water;
2. Stir in garlic, onion and fresh herbs and cook until fish is cooked through. Serve garnished with parsley.

Nutritional Information per Serving:
Calories: 104; Total Fat: 1.2 g; Carbs: 3.7 g; Dietary Fiber: 0.4 g; Sugars: 1.1 g; Protein: 19 g; Cholesterol: 49 mg; Sodium: 42 mg

49. Marinara Chicken

Yield: 1 Servings

Total Time: 75 Minutes

Prep Time: 10 Minutes

Cook Time: 65 Minutes

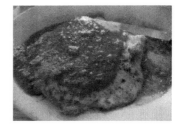

Ingredients
- 3 ounces boneless skinless chicken breast
- 1 small tomato, diced
- 2 cloves garlic
- 1 teaspoon oregano
- 1 teaspoon basil
- ½ teaspoon chili powder
- Dash garlic powder
- Dash pepper

Directions:
1. Preheat oven to 350°F.
2. Add half of diced tomatoes in a casserole dish.
3. Sprinkle chicken with garlic powder, salt and pepper and sear in pan for about 1-2 minutes per side; transfer to a dish with tomatoes and top with minced garlic.
4. Toss together the remaining ingredients in a small bowl and pour over chicken; bake, covered with aluminum foil, for about 45-60 minutes. Serve warm.

Nutritional Information per Serving:
Calories: 197; Total Fat: 6.9 g; Carbs: 7.5 g; Dietary Fiber: 2.4 g; Sugars:2.7 g; Protein: 26.2 g; Cholesterol: 76 mg; Sodium: 92 mg

50. Lemon Garlic Salmon

Yields: 4 Servings

Total Time: 35 Minutes

Prep Time: 15 Minutes

Cook Time: 30 Minutes

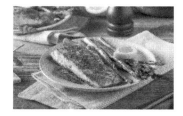

Ingredients

- 1 teaspoon extra virgin olive oil
- 4 salmon fillets
- 3 tablespoons freshly squeezed lemon juice
- 1 tablespoon coconut milk
- 1 teaspoon ground pepper
- 1 teaspoon dried parsley flakes
- 1 finely chopped clove garlic

Directions

1. Preheat your oven to 190°C (275°F). Coat a baking dish with extra virgin olive oil.

2. Rinse the fish under water and pat dry with paper towels.

Arrange the fish fillet in the coated baking dish and drizzle with lemon juice and coconut oil.

3. Sprinkle with ground pepper, parsley and garlic.

4. Bake in the oven for about 30 minutes or until the flakes easily when touched with a fork.

Nutritional Information per Serving:

Calories: 248; Total Fat: 12g; Carbs: 0.7g; Dietary Fiber: trace; Protein: 34.8g; Cholesterol: 0mg; Sodium: 82mg; trace

The Dinner Recipes

51. Gingery Roasted Chicken

Yield: 8 Servings

Total Time: 1 Hour 40 Minutes

Prep Time: 10 Minutes

Cook Time: 1Hour 30 Minutes

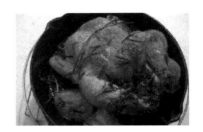

Ingredients:

- 1 tablespoon extra-virgin olive oil
- ½ cup apple cider vinegar
- 3 cloves garlic, minced
- 2-3 tablespoons minced ginger
- 3 pound whole chicken
- 1 pound chopped carrots
- handful of rosemary
- Pinch of sea salt
- Pinch of pepper

Directions:

1. Preheat oven to 400°F.

2. Place chicken in a baking dish. In a bowl, whisk together olive oil, apple cider vinegar, garlic, and ginger

until well combined; pour over the chicken and top with carrots and rosemary.

3. Sprinkle with salt and pepper and roast for about 1 ½ hours or until chicken is cooked through. Serve warm.

Nutritional Information per Serving:

Calories: 372; Total Fat: 14.6 g; Carbs: 7.6 g; Dietary Fiber: 1.7 g; Sugars: 3.3 g; Protein: 50 g; Cholesterol: 151 mg; Sodium: 220 mg

52. Tangerine Ham with Baby Carrots

Yield: 3 Servings

Total Time: 4.5 Hours

Prep Time: 30 Minutes

Cook Time: 4 Hours

Ingredients
- 1 (8 to 10-pound) smoked ham, bone-in, skin on
- 2 cups tangerine juice
- 2 tangerines, sliced thin, seeds removed
- 1 cup (2 sticks) unsalted butter, cut in chunks
- 1/4 cup extra-virgin olive oil
- 2 teaspoons liquid stevia
- 11/2 pounds carrots, peeled
- 2 cinnamon sticks
- 1/4 tsp. whole cloves
- 1 cup water

- 1 bunch fresh sage
- Sea salt & black pepper

Directions

1. Preheat oven to 300°F.

2. Place ham, fat-side down, in a roasting pan. Score the ham with ½-inch deep cuts across the skin, 2-inches apart with a sharp knife. Season with salt and pepper.

3. In a small bowl, mix oil and chopped sage leaves to make a paste; rub over the ham and bake for about 2 hours.

4. Meanwhile, make the glaze: set a large saucepan over medium heat; add tangerine juice, tangerines, butter, spices, stevia and water. Cook the mixture for about 40 minutes or until it forms a syrupy glaze.

5. After two hours of cooking ham, pour the tangerine glaze over it and scatter fruit pieces over it with the remaining sage leaves. Continue cooking for about 1 ½ hours more, basting with juices every 30 minutes.

6. Scatter the ham with carrots and continue cooking for 30 minutes more or until ham is dark and crispy and carrots are tender. Remove from oven and let cool before carving.

7. Serve with tangerine and carrot glaze on side.

Nutrition info Per Serving:
Calories: 362; Total Fat: 20.8 g; Carbs: 17.2 g; Dietary Fiber: 4.3 g; Sugars: 7 g; Protein: 26 g; Cholesterol: 102 mg; Sodium: 2074 mg

53. Pepper Crusted Steak

Yield: 1 Serving

Total Time: 15 Minutes

Prep Time: 10 Minutes

Cook Time: 5 Minutes

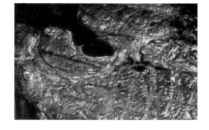

Ingredients
- 100 grams lean steak
- Dash of Worcestershire sauce
- Pinch of salt & pepper

Directions:
1. Pound meat until tender and flat; rub with salt and pepper and cook on high heat for about 3-5 minutes.

2. Serve topped with Worcestershire sauce and garnished with caramelized onions.

Nutritional Information per Serving:
Calories: 189; Total Fat: 6.2 g; Carbs: 0.2 g; Dietary Fiber: 0 g; Sugars: 0.1 g; Protein: 30.4 g; Cholesterol: 89 mg; Sodium: 228 mg

54. Tasty Sesame Salmon

Yield: 3 Servings

Total Time: 30 Minutes

Prep Time: 5 Minutes

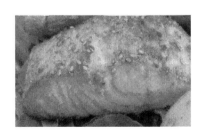

Cook Time: 25 Minutes

Ingredients
- 1 teaspoon dried chili flakes
- 1 teaspoon minced ginger root
- 2 tablespoon rice vinegar
- 2 tablespoons soy sauce
- 1 large clove garlic, minced
- 3 skinless wild salmon fillets
- 3 tablespoons white sesame seeds

Directions

1. In a zip-top bag, mix chili flakes, ginger, rice vinegar, soy sauce, and garlic; add salmon filets in the bag and refrigerate for at least 1 hour.

2. Preheat oven to 375°F.

3. Sprinkle sesame seeds onto a plate into a single layer; arrange the filets, face down, in the sesame seeds and transfer the fish onto a baking sheet lined with baking paper;

4. Sprinkle with more sesame seeds and bake for about 20 minutes.

5. Switch the oven to broil the fish for about 5 minutes or until sesame seeds are toasted.

Nutrition info Per Serving:
Calories: 248; Total Fat: 11 g; Carbs: 0.9 g; Dietary Fiber: 4 g; Sugars: 17.6 g; Protein: 35.2 g; Cholesterol: 78 mg; Sodium: 680 mg

55. Buffalo Chicken Fingers

Yield: 1 Serving

Total Time: 25 Minutes

Prep Time: 10 Minutes

Cook Time: 15 Minutes

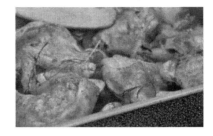

Ingredients
- 100 grams chicken, sliced into strips
- 4 tablespoons fresh lemon juice
- 2 tablespoons hot sauce
- Bread crumbs
- Pinch of salt & black pepper

Directions:
1. Marinate chicken in fresh lemon juice and salt for a few hours and then coat with crushed crumbs;

2. Fry in a pan until cooked through and browned.

3. Toss with black pepper and hot sauce and serve with raw celery, garnished with parsley.

Nutritional Information per Serving:
Calories: 169; Total Fat: 3.6 g; Carbs: 1.8 g; Dietary Fiber: 0.4 g; Sugars:1.6 g; Protein: 29.6g; Cholesterol: 77 mg; Sodium: 869 mg

56. Tasty Baked Chicken

Yield: 4 Servings

Total Time: 15 Minutes

Prep Time: 10 Minutes

Cook Time: 5 Minutes

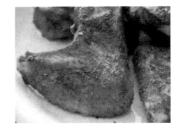

Ingredients
- 12 ounces boneless skinless chicken breast
- 1 packet stevia
- Rosemary
- Thyme
- Dash of sea salt
- Dash of pepper

Directions:
1. In a plastic bag, combine all ingredients; seal and shake thoroughly. Grill for about 5 minutes.

Nutritional Information per Serving:
Calories: 162; Total Fat: 6.3 g; Carbs: 0 g; Dietary Fiber: 0 g; Sugars: 0 g; Protein: 24.6 g; Cholesterol: 76 mg; Sodium: 132 mg

57. Tasty Grilled salmon

Yield: 4 Servings

Total Time: 25 Minutes

Prep Time: 15 Minutes

Cook Time: 10 Minutes

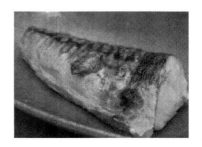

Ingredients

- 4 green olives, chopped
- 4 salmon fillets, each 5 ounces
- 2 tbsp. freshly squeezed lemon juice
- 1 tbsp. minced garlic
- 1 tbsp. chopped fresh parsley
- 4 tbsp. chopped fresh basil
- Cracked black pepper
- 4 thin slices lemon

Directions

1. Lightly coat grill rack with olive oil cooking spray and position it 4 inches from heat; heat grill to medium high.

2. Combine lemon juice, minced garlic, parsley and basil in a small bowl.

3. Coat fish with extra virgin olive oil and season with sea salt and pepper.

4. Top each fish fillet with equal amount of garlic mixture and place on the heated grill, herb-side down.

5. Grill over high heat for about 4 minutes or until the edges turn white; turn over and transfer the fish to aluminum foil.

6. Reduce heat and continue grilling for about 4 minutes more.

7. Transfer the grilled fish to serving plates and garnish with lemon slices and green olives. Serve immediately.

Nutritional Information Per Serving:

Calories: 241; Total Fat: 11.1 g; Carbs: 1 g; Dietary Fiber: trace; Sugars: trace; Protein: 34.8 g; Cholesterol: 78 mg; Sodium: 81 mg

58. **Spiced Chicken Patties**

Yield: 1 Serving

Total Time: 40 Minutes

Prep Time: 10 Minutes

Cook Time: 30 Minutes

Ingredients
- 100 grams ground chicken breast
- 1 clove garlic, minced
- ½ red onion, minced
- Dash of garlic powder
- Dash of onion powder
- Pinch of cayenne pepper
- Pinch of salt & pepper

Directions:

1. In a small bowl, mix all ingredients until well combined; form three patties and fry in a saucepan, deglazing with water to keep chicken moist.

2. Cook until chicken is cooked through and serve.

Nutritional Information per Serving:

Calories: 114; Total Fat: 0.9 g; Carbs: 1.6 g; Dietary Fiber: 0.4 g; Sugars: 0.6 g; Protein: 25.2 g; Cholesterol: 63 mg; Sodium: 50 mg

59. Scrumptious Shrimp

Yield: 1 Serving

Total Time: 30 Minutes

Prep Time: 10 Minutes

Cook Time: 20 Minutes

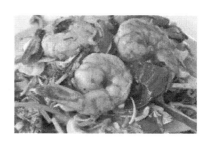

Ingredients
- 3 ounces shrimp, diced
- 5 tablespoons vegetable broth
- 1 clove garlic, minced
- 3 ounces shredded cabbage
- Dash of Chinese 5 Spice
- dash of onion powder
- ½ packet stevia
- Pinch of salt & pepper

Directions:
1. Add a tablespoon of broth to a pan and sauté garlic; stir in cabbage and two tablespoons of broth.

2. Cook over medium heat for a few minutes; transfer cabbage to a plate while still crunchy and stir the remaining ingredients in the pan; stir fry and return cabbage. Cook for about 1-2 minutes.

Nutritional Information per Serving:
Calories: 140: Total Fat: 2 g; Carbs: 7.8 g; Dietary Fiber: 2.2 g; Sugars: 3.1 g; Protein: 22.2 g; Cholesterol: 179 mg; Sodium: 696 mg

60. Ground Beef Tacos

Yield: 1 Serving

Total Time: 35 Minutes

Prep Time: 10 Minutes

Cook Time: 25 Minutes

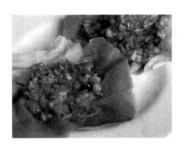

Ingredients
- 100 grams lean ground beef
- 1 clove garlic, minced
- ½ red onion, minced
- Lettuce leaves
- Cayenne pepper
- Fresh chopped cilantro
- Pinch of dried oregano
- Dash of onion powder
- Dash of garlic powder
- Pinch of salt & pepper

Directions:
1. Fry beef in a splash of lemon juice until browned;

2. Add garlic, onion and spices, and water and simmer for about 5-10 minutes.

3. Season with salt and serve taco style in romaine lettuce or butter lettuce or with a side of salsa or tomatoes.

Nutritional Information per Serving:
Calories: 194; Total Fat: 6.3 g; Carbs: 1.9 g; Dietary Fiber: 0.5 g; Sugars: 0.7 g; Protein: 30.6 g; Cholesterol: 89 mg; Sodium: 67 mg

61. Poached Halibut

Yield: 1 Serving

Total Time: 20 Minutes

Prep Time: 10 Minutes

Cook Time: 10 Minutes

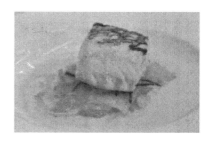

Ingredients
- 100 grams halibut
- 1 clove garlic, minced
- 1 tablespoon chopped red onion
- ½ teaspoon fresh ginger
- 1 tablespoon fresh lemon juice
- Pinch of grated orange zest
- ½ cup vegetable broth
- Pinch of salt & pepper
- Pinch of stevia

Directions:
1. In a pan, heat broth and stir in garlic, onion, lemon juice, and spices; poach fish for about 5-10 minutes or until cooked through. Serve topped with cooking juices.

Nutritional Information per Serving:
Calories: 121; Total Fat: 2.4 g; Carbs: 2.7 g; Dietary Fiber: 0.6 g; Sugars: 1.1 g; Protein: 21.5 g; Cholesterol: 211 mg; Sodium: 542 mg

62. Crock Pot Coconut Curry Shrimp

Yield: 8 Servings

Total Time: 2 Hours 5 Minutes

Prep Time: 5 Minutes

Cook Time: 2 Hours

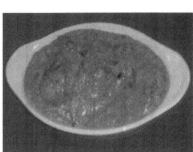

Ingredients

- 1 pound shrimp, with shells
- 15 ounces water
- 30 ounces light coconut milk
- ½ cup Thai red curry sauce
- ¼ cup cilantro
- 2½ teaspoon lemon garlic seasoning

Directions

1. In a slow cooker, combine water, coconut milk, red curry paste, cilantro, and lemon garlic seasoning;

2. Stir to mix well and cook on high for about 2 hours.

3. Add shrimp and continue cooking for another 30 minutes or until shrimp is cooked through.

4. Serve garnished with cilantro.

Nutrition info Per Serving:

Calories: 312; Total Fat: 26.3 g; Carbs: 6.8 g; Dietary Fiber: 2.3 g; Sugars: 3.5 g; Protein: 15.3 g; Cholesterol: 119 mg; Sodium: 156 mg

63. Beef Stir Fry w/ Red Onions & Peppers

Yield: 4 Servings

Total Time: 20 Minutes

Prep Time: 10 Minutes

Cook Time: 10 Minutes

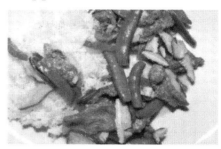

Ingredients:

- 1 pound grass-fed flank steak, thinly sliced strips
- 1 tablespoon rice wine
- 2 teaspoons balsamic vinegar
- Pinch of sea salt
- pinch of pepper
- 3 teaspoons extra-virgin olive oil
- 1 large yellow onion, thinly chopped
- 1/2 red bell pepper, thinly sliced
- 1/2 green bell pepper, thinly sliced
- 1 tablespoon toasted sesame seeds
- 1 teaspoon crushed red pepper flakes

Directions:

1. Place meat in a bowl; stir in rice wine and vinegar, sea salt and pepper. Toss to coat well.

2. Heat a tablespoon of olive oil in a pan set over medium high heat; add meat and cook for about 1 minute or until meat is browned;

3. Stir for another 2 minutes and then remove from heat.

4. Heat the remaining oil to the pan and sauté onions for about 2 minutes or until caramelized;

5. Stir in pepper and cook for 2 minutes more; return meat to pan and stir in sesame seeds and red pepper flakes. Serve hot!

Nutritional Information per Serving:

Calories: 296; Total Fat: 14.3 g; Carbs: 8.3 g; Dietary Fiber: 1.6 g; Sugars: 4.2 g; Protein: 32.76 g; Cholesterol: 62 mg; Sodium: 157 mg

64. Ginger Chicken with Veggies

Yields: 4 Servings

Total Time: 15 Minutes

Prep Time: 10 Minutes

Cook Time: 5 Minutes

Ingredients

- 2 cup skinless, boneless, and cooked chicken breast meat, diced
- ¼ cup extra virgin olive and canola oil mixture
- 1 teaspoon powdered ginger
- ½ red onion, sliced
- 2 cloves garlic, minced
- ½ bell pepper, sliced
- 1 cup thinly sliced carrots
- ½ cup finely chopped celery

- 1 cup chicken broth (not salted)

Directions

1. Add the oil mixture to a skillet set over medium heat; sauté onion and garlic until translucent.

2. Stir in the remaining ingredients and simmer for a few minutes or until the veggies are tender.

Nutrition Information per Serving:

Calories: 425; Total Fat: 21.1 g; Carbs: 6.5 g; Dietary Fiber: 1.5 g; Sugars: 3.1 g Protein: 52 g; Cholesterol: 130 mg; Sodium: 301 mg

65. Chili Fried Steak with Toasted Cashews

Yields: 4 Servings

Total Time: 35 Minutes

Prep Time: 10 Minutes

Cook Time: 25 Minutes

Ingredients

- ½ tbsp. extra virgin olive oil or canola oil
- 1 pound sliced lean beef
- 2 tablespoons apple cider vinegar
- 2 teaspoon fish sauce
- 2 teaspoons red curry paste
- 1 cup green capsicum, diced
- 24 toasted cashews

- 1 teaspoon arrowroot
- 1 teaspoon liquid stevia
- ½ cup water

Directions

1. Add oil to a pan set over medium heat; add beef and fry until it is no longer pink inside. Stir in red curry paste and cook for a few more minutes.

2. Stir in stevia, vinegar, fish sauce, capsicum and water; simmer for about 10 minutes.

3. Mix cooked arrowroot with water to make a paste; stir the paste into the sauce to thicken it.

4. Remove the pan from heat and add toasted cashews. Serve.

Nutrition Information per Serving:

Calories: 252; Total Fat: 9.7 g; Carbs: 4 g; Dietary Fiber: 0.6 g; Sugars: 2.1 g Protein: 35.1 g; Cholesterol: 101 mg; Sodium: 441 mg

66. **Tasty Coconut Cod**

Yields: 4 Servings

Total Time: 35 Minutes

Prep Time: 25 Minutes

Cook Time: 10 Minutes

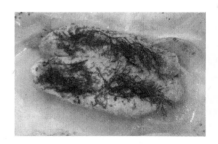

Ingredients:

- 24 ounces cod fillets, sliced into small strips
- 2 tablespoons coconut oil
- 1 cup finely shredded coconut
- 2 cups coconut milk
- 1 ½ cups coconut flour
- ¼ teaspoon sea salt
- 1 ½ teaspoon ginger powder

Directions

1. Rinse and debone the fish fillets.

2. In a bowl, combine ginger powder, coconut flour and sea salt; set aside.

3. Add coconut milk to another bowl and set aside.

4. Add shredded coconut to another bowl and set aside.

5. Dip the fillets into coconut milk, then into the flour mixture, back into the milk, and finally into shredded coconut.

6. Add coconut oil to a skillet set over high heat; when melted and hot, add the fish fillets and cook for about 5 minutes per side or until cooked through.

Nutrition Information per Serving:

Calories: 609; Total Fat: 44.3 g; Carbs: 13.2 g; Dietary Fiber: 6.4 g; Sugars: 5.7 g Protein: 43.1 g; Cholesterol: 34 mg; Sodium: 283 mg

67. Grilled Chicken with Fresh Herb Marinade

Yield: 4 Servings

Total Time: 40 Minutes

Prep Time: 10 Minutes

Cook Time: 30 Minutes

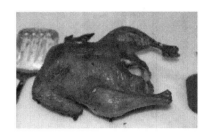

Ingredients

- 1 cup chopped mixed fresh herb leaves (basil, parsley, cilantro)
- 2 large garlic cloves, chopped
- 1/4 cup apple cider vinegar
- 1/4 cup extra-virgin olive oil
- 3 teaspoons sea salt
- 1/4 teaspoon pepper
- 1 pound chicken breasts, boneless, skinless, sliced in half lengthwise

Directions

1. In a food processor, process together herbs, garlic, vinegar, oil, salt and pepper until smooth; transfer to a Ziploc bag and add chicken.

2. Shake to coat chicken well and refrigerate for about 30 minutes; grill the chicken for about 15 minutes per side or until cooked through.

Nutrition Information per Serving:

Calories: 183; Total Fat: 8 g; Carbs: 1 g; Dietary Fiber: 0 g; Sugars: 0 g Protein: 26 g; Cholesterol: 65 mg; Sodium: 73 mg

68. Orange-Cranberry Crusted Salmon

Yield: 4 Servings

Total Time: 15 Minutes

Prep Time: 15 Minutes

Cook Time: 0 Minutes

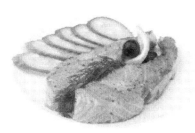

Ingredients

- Olive oil cooking spray
- 4 salmon filets
- Salt & pepper to taste
- 2 tablespoons extra virgin olive oil
- ¼ cup dried cranberries, chopped
- ½ cup walnuts, chopped
- 1 teaspoon orange zest
- 1 tablespoon Dijon mustard
- 2 tablespoons parsley, chopped

Directions

1. Preheat your oven to 370°F.

2. Lightly coat a baking sheet with olive oil cooking spray. Generously season the fish filets with sea salt and pepper and arrange them on the baking sheet.

3. Mix the remaining ingredients in a small bowl until well blended; press onto the filets and bake in the reheated oven for about 20 minutes or until the topping is lightly browned.

4. Remove from oven and serve.

Nutritional Information Per Serving:

Calories: 400; Total Fat: 27.4 g; Carbs: 2.6 g; Dietary Fiber: 1.6 g; Protein: 38.5 g; Cholesterol: 78 mg; Sodium: 124 mg

69. Grilled Chicken & Green Onion

Yield: 1 Serving

Total Time: 15 Minutes

Prep Time: 10 Minutes

Cook Time: 5 Minutes

Ingredients
- 3 ounces chicken breast
- 1 green onion, chopped
- Pinch of garlic powder
- Pinch of sea salt
- Pinch of pepper

Directions:
Place chicken on grill and top with onion slices; sprinkle with garlic powder, salt and pepper and grill for about 5 minutes or until chicken is cooked through.

Nutritional Information per Serving:
Calories: 176; Total Fat: 6.3 g; Carbs: 3.4 g; Dietary Fiber: 0.8 g; Sugars: 1.5 g; Protein: 5 g; Cholesterol: 76 mg; Sodium: 61 mg

70. Shrimp Salad w/ Grapefruit and Avocado

Yield: 2 Servings

Total Time: 20 Minutes

Prep Time: 10 Minutes

Cook Time: 10 Minutes

Ingredients

- 2 tablespoons chili oil
- 1 cup shrimp
- ½ teaspoon salt
- ½ teaspoon pepper
- 1 avocado, cubed
- 1 grapefruit, cubed
- ¼ cup lemon juice

Directions

1. Heat chili oil in a saucepan set over medium heat; add shrimp and cook until opaque and lightly browned.

2. Remove the pan from heat and season shrimp with sea salt and pepper.

3. In a serving bowl, pack avocado slices as tightly as possible, and then top with a layer of shrimp, grapefruit, and drizzle with lemon juice. Serve while shrimp are still hot!

Nutritional Information Per Serving

Calories: 488; Total Fat: 35.8 g; Carbs: 16.5 g; Dietary fiber: 7.7 g; Protein: 28.2 g; Cholesterol: 237 mg; Sodium: 868 mg

71. Chicken Stir-Fry

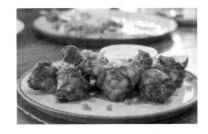

Yield: 4 Servings

Total Time: 30 Minutes

Prep Time: 10 Minutes

Cook time: 20 Minutes

Ingredients

- 4 chicken breasts (butterfly), marinate in egg white overnight
- 2 cups red pepper
- 2 cups mange tout
- 2 cups grated carrot
- 2 cups broccoli
- 2 cups almonds
- 2 cloves of garlic
- ½ tsp. ginger
- 2 tbsp. soya sauce
- 125ml chicken stock.
- 2 tbsp. coconut oil

Directions

1. Heat coconut oil in a pan over medium fire. Sauté the garlic and ginger until fragrant.

2. Cook the chicken breast in the oil and then add the vegetables. Toss and cook until almost done.

3. Add 2 tbsp. soya sauce and 125ml chicken stock. Allow to simmer uncovered until the broth evaporates.

Nutritional Information per Serving:

Calories: 186; Total Fat: 11 g; Carbs: 4 g; Dietary Fiber: 1.5 g; Sugars: 1.9 g; Protein: 17 g; Cholesterol: 550 mg; Sodium: 1272 mg

72. **Chicken and Mushroom Stew**

Yield: 4 Servings

Total Time: 60 Minutes

Prep Time: 10 Minutes

Cook Time: 50 Minutes

Ingredients

-
- 8 pcs. chicken thighs
- 4 tbsp. butter
- 3 cloves garlic, minced
- 6 cups mushrooms
- 1 cup chicken stock
- ½ tsp. dried thyme
- ½ tsp. dried oregano
- ½ tsp. dried basil
- ¼ cup heavy cream
- ½ cup parmesan cheese, grated
- 1 tbsp. whole-grain mustard

Directions

1. Preheat oven to 400F

2. Season chicken thighs with salt and pepper

3. Heat an oven-proof pan over medium fire and melt 2 tbsp. of butter.

4. Add the chicken, skin-side down, and fry both sides until golden brown, or about 2-3 minutes per side. Set aside.

5. Melt remaining 2 tbsp. butter. Add garlic, thyme, oregano and basil and mushrooms, and cook, stirring occasionally.

6. Cook until browned, about 5-6 minutes, season with salt and pepper, to taste.

7. Stir in chicken stock, then chicken back to the pan.

8. Pour everything into a baking dish with the chicken.

9. Place into oven and roast until completely cooked through for about 25-30 minutes. Set aside chicken.

10. Transfer sauces back into the original pan.

11. Stir in heavy cream, parmesan cheese and mustard. Bring to a boil; reduce heat and simmer until slightly reduced, about 5 minutes.

12. Serve chicken immediately, topped with mushroom mixture.

Nutritional Information per Serving:

Calories: 203; Total Fat: 3 g; Carbs: 9 g; Dietary Fiber: 1.5 g; Sugars: 2.9 g; Protein: 28 g; Cholesterol: 550 mg; Sodium: 272 mg

73. Bacon, Beef Sausage and Broccoli Casserole

Yield: 4 Servings

Total Time: 45 Minutes

Prep Time: 10 Minutes

Cook time: 35 Minutes

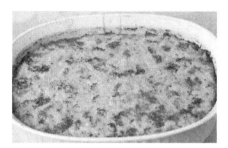

Ingredients

- 500 g beef sausage
- 1/2 head of broccoli
- 8 slices of bacon
- 1/2 cup of cream
- 1 tbsp. Dijon mustard
- 100 g grated cheddar cheese

Directions

1. Preheat oven to 350F

2. Slice the sausage and place in a small baking dish.

3. Slice the bacon and add to the sausage.

4. Break the broccoli into florets and arrange between the meat.

5. Mix the cream and mustard in a bowl and pour it all over the casserole, then top with the cheese.

6. Bake in the oven for 35 minutes.

Nutritional Information per Serving:

Calories: 300; Total Fat: 25 g; Carbs: 3 g; Dietary Fiber: 0.7 g; Sugars: 1.8 g; Protein: 20.7 g; Cholesterol: 56 mg; Sodium: 272 mg

74. Herbed London Broil

Yield: 1 Serving

Total Time: 40 Minutes

Prep Time: 10 Minutes

Cook Time: 30 Minutes

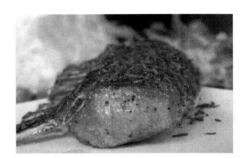

Ingredients
- 100 grams lean London broil,
- sliced thinly into strips
- 1 clove garlic, minced
- 1 red onion, minced
- ¼ cup beef broth or water
- Chopped Italian parsley
- Pinch of rosemary
- 1/8 teaspoon thyme
- Pinch of salt & pepper

Directions:
1. Coat beef with salt and pepper and add to a pan along with beef broth and
2. herbs; cook until beef is cooked through.
3. Serve garnished with parsley.

Nutritional Information per Serving:

Calories: 201; Total Fat: 6.6 g; Carbs: 1.4 g; Dietary Fiber: 0.4 g; Sugars:0.6 g; Protein: 31.7 g; Cholesterol: 89 mg; Sodium: 257 mg

75. **Tasty Oregano Chicken**

Yield: 1 Serving

Total Time: 30 Minutes

Prep Time: 10 Minutes

Cook Time: 20 Minutes

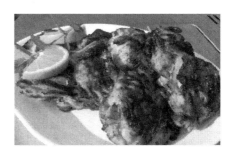

Ingredients
- 100 grams chicken breast
- ¼ cup chicken broth
- 1 teaspoon dried oregano
- ¼ teaspoon onion powder
- ¼ teaspoon garlic powder
- Pinch of salt & pepper
- ½ cup bread crumbs

Directions:
1. Mix dry spices with crumbs; dip chicken in broth and dust with Melba mix.

2. Add t a baking dish and add the remaining broth; bake in a 350°F oven for about 15-20 minutes or until browned and crusty.

Nutritional Information per Serving:
Calories: 133; Total Fat: 3 g; Carbs: 2.3 g; Dietary Fiber: 0.8 g; Sugars:0.6 g; Protein: 22.8 g; Cholesterol: 64 mg; Sodium: 243 mg

76. Tasty Citric Chicken

Yield: 1 Serving

Total Time: 40 Minutes

Prep Time: 10 Minutes

Cook Time: 30 Minutes

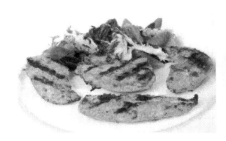

Ingredients
- 100 grams chicken breast
- ½ red onion, minced
- Juice of ½ lemon
- Pinch of lemon zest
- Pinch of saffron
- Pinch of ground coriander
- Pinch of ginger
- Pinch of salt & pepper
- Lemon slices

Directions:
1. Soak saffron in fresh lemon juice; crush into paste and then add dry spices.

2. Dip in chicken and rub remaining spices into chicken; sprinkle with salt and pepper and wrap in foil;

3. Place in baking dish and cover with lemon slices and saffron mi. bake in a 350°F oven for about 20-30 minutes or until chicken is cooked through.

Nutritional Information per Serving:
Calories: 122; Total Fat: 2.6 g; Carbs: 1.9 g; Dietary Fiber: 0.5 g; Sugars:0.6 g; Protein: 21.4 g; Cholesterol: 64 mg; Sodium: 52 mg

77. Healthy Stuffed Mushrooms

Yield: 4 Servings

Total Time: 20 Minutes

Prep Time: 10 Minutes

Cook Time: 10 Minutes

Ingredients

- 1 cup parsley, chopped
- 1 teaspoon lemon juice
- 1 clove garlic, chopped
- ½ cup pine nuts
- ½ cup sun dried tomatoes
- ¼ teaspoon sea salt
- ¼ cup extra virgin olive oil
- 1 package (8 ounce) mushrooms

Directions

1. Pulse parsley in a food processor until well chopped.

2. Add lemon juice, garlic, pine nuts, sundried tomatoes and salt and continue pulsing until smooth.

3. Add extra virgin olive oil and pulse to blend well.

4. Remove the stems from mushrooms; stuff each with pesto and bake at 350°F for about 10 minutes.

Nutritional Information per Serving:

Calories: 271; Total Fat: 26.5 g; Carbs: 8.5 g; Dietary Fiber: 2.5 g; Protein: 5.3 g; Cholesterol: 0 mg; Sodium: 166 mg; Sugars: 1.8 g

The Snacks Recipes

78. **Roasted Chili-Vinegar Peanuts**

Yield: 4 Servings

Total Time: 15 Minutes

Prep Time: 5 Minutes

Cook Time: 10 Minutes

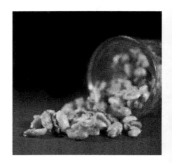

Ingredients

- 1 tablespoon coconut oil
- 2 cups raw peanuts, unsalted
- 2 teaspoon sea salt
- 2 tablespoon apple cider vinegar
- 1 teaspoon chili powder
- 1 teaspoon fresh lime zest

Directions

1. Preheat oven to 350°F.

2. In a large bowl, toss together coconut oil, peanuts, and salt until well coated; transfer to a rimmed baking sheet and roast in the oven for about 15 minutes or until fragrant.

3. Transfer the roasted peanuts to a bowl and add vinegar, chili powder and lime zest; toss to coat well and serve.

Nutritional Information per Serving:

Calories: 447; Total Fat: 39.5g; Carbs: 12.3 g; Dietary Fiber: 6.5 g; Sugars: 3 g; Protein: 18.9 g; Cholesterol: 0 mg; Sodium: 956 mg

79. Tahini Hummus (Nut-Free, Vegan, Vegetarian, Gluten-Free)

Yield: 4 Servings

Total Time: 20 Minutes

Prep Time: 10 Minutes

Cook Time: 10 Minutes

Ingredients

- 2 tablespoons extra-virgin olive oil
- 1/4 cup toasted sesame tahini
- 1/4 cup apple cider vinegar
- 1 cup chickpeas
- 1 clove garlic, minced
- 1/2 teaspoon ground cumin
- 1 teaspoon sea salt
- 3 tablespoons water

Directions

In a food processor, combine all ingredients and pulse until very smooth. Serve with carrots or cucumber slices.

Nutritional Information per Serving:

Calories: 168; Total Fat: 9.1 g; Carbs: 17 g; Dietary Fiber: 5.1 g; Sugars: 2.8 g; Protein: 6.2 g; Cholesterol: 0 mg; Sodium: 249 mg

80. Baked Beet Chips with Tzatziki

Yield: 2 Servings

Total Time: 40 Minutes

Prep Time: 10 Minutes

Cook Time: 30 Minutes

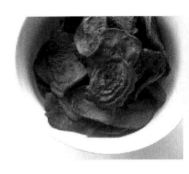

Ingredients

- 5 beets, peeled and very thinly sliced
- 3 tbsp. palm oil
- Coarse sea salt

Tzatziki:

- 1 ¼ cups coconut yogurt
- ¾ cup cucumber, peeled and minced finely
- 1 clove garlic, minced
- ½ tbsp. fresh parsley, minced
- ½ tbsp. dill
- ½ tbsp. chives, minced
- ½ tbsp. fresh mint leaves, minced
- 1 tsp freshly squeezed lemon juice
- ½ tsp coarse sea salt
- Freshly ground pepper

Directions

1. Start by preheating your oven to 325 F and line a rimmed baking sheet with parchment paper

2. Lay out the sliced beets on a paper towel, to absorb most of the moisture so they can cook faster.

3. Transfer the sliced beets on the baking sheet and liberally coat with palm oil or your favorite oil. Use your hands to ensure all the slices are well coated.

4. Lightly grease another baking sheet and place it over the beets, this will help them cook flat and evenly.

5. Bake the sliced beets for about 20 minutes at center rack, rotating halfway through. Remove the top baking sheet and bake uncovered for another 10 minutes until slightly browned.

6. Remove from oven and let cool and become crisp.

Tzatziki:

Combine all the ingredients until you get an even consistency. If it's too thick, add a little water to thin. Serve as a dip for the beet chips. Enjoy!

Nutritional Information per Serving:

Calories: 377; Total Fat: 23.4 g; Carbs: 18.1 g; Dietary Fiber: 5.6 g; Sugars: 29.5 g; Protein: 8.2 g; Cholesterol: 0 mg; Sodium: 917 mg

81. Dry-Roasted Chickpea (Nut-Free, Vegan, Vegetarian, Gluten-Free)

Yield: 6 Servings

Total Time: 54 Minutes

Prep Time: 10 Minutes

Cook Time: 44 Minutes

Ingredients

- 2 cups chickpeas
- 2 teaspoons extra-virgin olive oil
- 1/4 teaspoon salt
- ¼ teaspoon black pepper

Directions

1. Preheat oven to 425°F. Spread chickpeas in a medium baking dish and pat them dry with paper towel; bake, stirring halfway through, for about 22 minutes.

2. Transfer to a large bowl and toss with olive oil, sea salt and pepper; return to oven and bake, stirring hallway through, for another 22 minutes or until dry and golden.

Nutritional Information per Serving:

Calories: 256; Total Fat: 5.6 g; Carbs: 19.5 g; Dietary Fiber: 11.6 g; Sugars: 7.1 g; Protein: 12.9 g; Cholesterol: 0 mg; Sodium: 113 mg

82. Bacon-Avocado stuffed Peppers

Yield: 4 Servings

Total Time: 30 Minutes

Prep Time: 10 Minutes

Cook Time: 20 Minutes

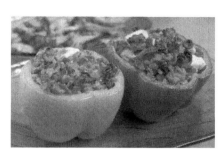

Ingredients

1. 450g sweet baby peppers
2. 150g bacon, chopped
3. 2 ripe avocados
4. 1 tbsp. hot sauce
5. 2 tbsp. freshly squeezed lime juice
6. ½ bunch cilantro, chopped
7. Coarse sea salt

Directions

1. Preheat your oven to 350 F.

2. Cut the peppers in half, lengthwise, removing the seeds and membrane. Arrange them in a baking sheet and lightly spray with cooking spray and bake for 10 minutes.

3. As the peppers are baking, mash up the avocado in a bowl and combine with the lime juice, hot sauce, salt and the cilantro and sauté the bacon in a skillet until they become crisp and browned.

4. Use a spoon to scoop the avocado mash into the peppers and top with bacon bits. Enjoy!

Nutritional Information per Serving:

Calories: 431; Total Fat: 35.5 g; Carbs: 17.5 g; Dietary Fiber: 8.7 g; Sugars: 3.3 g; Protein: 16.8 g; Cholesterol: 41 mg; Sodium: 971 mg

83. Healthy Seed Crackers (Nut-Free, Vegan, Vegetarian, Gluten-Free)

Yield: 6 Servings

Total Time: 1 Hour 5 Minutes

Prep Time: 5 Minutes

Cook Time: 1 Hour

Ingredients

- 1 teaspoon sea salt
- 1/2 cup raw buckwheat
- 1/2 cup linseeds
- 1 1/2 cups sunflower seeds
- 1/4 cup chia seeds
- 1 1/2 cups warm water

Directions

1. Mix together all ingredients in a large bowl; set aside for about 20 minutes, stirring occasionally.

2. Preheat oven to 325°F.

3. Press the mixture into a baking tray lined with baking paper and bake for about 1 hours or until golden and crisp. Remove from oven and cut into pieces. Enjoy!

Nutritional Information per Serving:

Calories: 199; Total Fat: 12.1 g; Carbs: 16.9 g; Dietary Fiber: 8 g; Sugars: 0.3 g; Protein: 7.4 g; Cholesterol: 0 mg; Sodium: 321 mg

84. Tasty Candied Pecans

Yield: 4 Servings

Total Time: 30 Minutes

Prep Time: 15 Minutes

Cook Time: 15 Minutes

Ingredients

- ½ cup pecans
- 2 tablespoons maple syrup
- 1 tablespoon extra-virgin olive oil
- ½ teaspoon sea salt

Directions

1. In a bowl, toss together all ingredients and spread into a baking dish. Bake at 350°F for about 15 minutes.

2. Remove from oven and let cool before serving.

Nutritional Information per Serving:

Calories: 315; Total Fat: 30.3 g; Carbs: 12.1 g; Dietary Fiber: 4 g; Protein: 4 g; Cholesterol: 0 mg; Sodium: 235 mg; Sugars: 7.3 g

85. Raw Protein-Packed Quinoa Energy Bars (Vegan, Vegetarian, Gluten-Free)

Yield: 4 Servings

Total Time: 25 Minutes

+Freezing Time

Prep Time: 10 Minutes

Cook Time: 5 Minutes

Ingredients

- 1 teaspoon coconut oil
- ½ cup rolled oats
- 1 cup quinoa, soaked overnight and drained
- ½ cup dried pitted dates
- ¼ cup pumpkin seeds
- ¼ cup sesame seeds
- ¼ cup sunflower seeds
- ½ cup almonds, crushed
- A pinch sea salt

Directions

1. Combine all ingredients in a food processor and pulse until smooth; spread onto a paper foil and cover with plastic wrap;

2. Roll into a 1-inch thin layer and freeze for about 1 hour; cut into bars and serve.

Nutritional Information per Serving:

Calories: 452; Total Fat: 20.3 g; Carbs: 17.7 g; Dietary Fiber: 8.9 g; Sugars: 14.9 g; Protein: 14.7 g; Cholesterol: 0 mg; Sodium: 65 mg

86. Healthy Roasted pumpkin seeds

Yield: 3 Servings

Total Time: 30 Minutes

Prep Time: 10 Minutes

Cook Time: 20 Minutes

Ingredients

- Scrape out the seed and pulp from 1 or 2 pumpkins
- Garlic salt
- ¼ cup salt
- 2-3 tbsp. olive oil

Directions

1. Soak the pulp and seeds in a bowl of water with the ¼ cup salt. Let stand for 2 days.

2. After the 2 days, separate the seeds from the pulp and set your oven to 325 F.

3. Rinse the seeds and pat dry with paper towels then sprinkle with garlic salt and coat with the olive oil. Line a baking sheet with parchment paper and spread out the seeds.

4. Roast for 20 minutes until they start browning. Remove from oven and let cool slightly. Enjoy!

87. Candied Macadamia Nuts

Yield: 2 Servings

Total Time: 25 Minutes

Prep Time: 10 Minutes

Cook Time: 15 Minutes

Ingredients

- 2 cups macadamia nuts
- 1 tablespoon extra-virgin olive oil
- 2 tablespoons   agave nectar or honey
- ½ teaspoon sea salt

Directions

1. In a bowl, toss together all ingredients and spread into a baking dish. Bake at 350°F for about 15 minutes or until browned.

2. Remove from oven and let cool before serving.

Nutritional Information per Serving:

Calories: 602; Total Fat: 58.9 g; Carbs: 18.3 g; Dietary Fiber: 5.9 g; Protein: 5.7 g; Cholesterol: 0 mg; Sodium: 436 mg; Sugars: 20.1 g

88. Barbequed Peaches & Plum with Cream Cheese

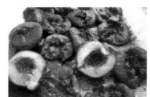

Yield: 4 Servings

Total Time: 25 Minutes

Prep Time: 15 Minutes

Cook Time: 10 Minutes

Ingredients:

- 10 ripe peaches, cut in halves and pitted
- 24 purple/ red plums cut in halves and pitted, with 4 sliced thinly
- 2 tbsp. freshly squeezed lemon juice
- 1 cup water
- ½ cup raw honey
- 6 tbsp. organic butter, melted
- Cream cheese for serving

Directions:

1. Prepare your grill and set to medium heat.

2. Meanwhile, place a medium saucepan over medium to high heat and add the water, sliced plums and ¾ cup of honey.

3. Once it starts boiling, cover and bring to a gentle simmer for 10 minutes. The plums should be super soft.

4. Place the cooked plums in your food processor and pulse until it forms a smooth puree. Scoop the puree into a small bowl and combine with lemon juice.

5. Now, whisk the melted butter with the remaining honey and set aside.

6. Grill the peaches and plums over medium heat until desired tenderness is achieved, that's about 6 minutes. Baste the fruits with the butter-honey paste and turn them

once on the grill. Keep grilling until they caramelize and char slightly say about 2 more minutes.

7. Serve the grilled fruits on fruit bowls and drizzle with the plum puree. Top with a generous dollop of cream cheese and enjoy!

Nutritional Information per Serving:

Calories: 306; Total Fat: 25.5 g; Carbs: 19.5 g; Dietary Fiber: 8.7 g; Sugars: 3.3 g; Protein: 16.8 g; Cholesterol: 41 mg; Sodium: 971 mg

89. Healthy Spinach Cake

Yield: 12 Spinach Cake Slices

(6 Servings)

Total Time: 25 Minutes

Prep Time: 15 Minutes

Cook Time: 10 Minutes

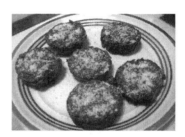

Ingredients

- 1 ½ pounds spinach, rinsed
- 1 cup pine nuts
- 2 cloves garlic, minced
- ½ cup currants
- 1 teaspoon sea salt
- 2 large eggs, whisked
- 3 tablespoons grapeseed oil

Directions

1. Wilt spinach in a pan set over low heat for about 5 minutes; drain and let cool a bit before squeezing moisture out of the spinach.

2. Pulse the spinach in a food processor until coarsely chopped; set aside.

3. Warm oil in a skillet; add pine nuts and sauté for a few minutes or until golden browned.

4. Stir in garlic and continue cooking for 1 more minute.

5. Combine the pine mixture, currants, blended spinach, eggs, and salt in a bowl; spread the mixture into a coated baking dish and bake at 350°F for about 35 minutes.

Nutritional Information per Serving:

Calories: 270; Total Fat: 22.2 g; Carbs: 8.9 g; Dietary Fiber: 2.9 g; Protein: 9.3 g; Cholesterol: 61 mg; Sodium: 313 mg; Sugars: 2.1 g

90. Grilled Pineapple Sundaes with Shredded Coconut

Yield: 2 Servings

Total Time: 20 Minutes

Prep Time: 10 Minutes

Cook Time: 10 Minutes

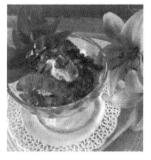

Ingredients:

- 1 whole ripe pineapple. Peeled, cored and cut in rings
- ½ cup shredded coconut, sweetened

- 2 tsp vegetable oil
- Frozen vanilla yogurt, fat free
- Mint sprigs

Directions:

1. Prepare a grill and set to medium.

2. Lightly brush the pineapple rings with vegetable oil and place on the grill.

3. Turn the pineapples once or twice and grill until they are soft and a bit charred, for about 8 minutes. Transfer the pineapples to a cutting board and chop them up.

4. Now toast the shredded coconut in a small pan over low heat and serve on a plate.

5. Serve the fro-yo (frozen yogurt) into sundae glasses or ice cream bowl and place the grilled pineapple on top, sprinkle with toasted coconut and garnish with mint sprigs. Serve immediately.

Nutritional Information per Serving:

Calories: 197; Total Fat: 11.3 g; Carbs: 18.4 g; Dietary Fiber: 3 g; Sugars: 15.3 g; Protein: 6.8 g; Cholesterol: 0 mg; Sodium: 28 mg

91. **Vinegar & Salt Kale Chips**

Yield: 2 Servings

Total Time: 22 Minutes

Prep Time: 10 Minutes

Cook Time: 12 Minutes

Ingredients

- 1 head kale, chopped
- 1 teaspoon extra virgin olive oil
- 1 tablespoon apple cider vinegar
- ½ teaspoon sea salt

Directions

1. Place kale in a bowl and drizzle with vinegar and extra virgin olive oil; sprinkle with salt and massage the ingredients with hands.

2. Spread the kale out onto two paper-lined baking sheets and bake at 375°F for about 12 minutes or until crispy.

3. Let cool for about 10 minutes before serving.

Nutritional Information per Serving:

Calories: 152; Total Fat: 8.2 g; Carbs: 15.2 g; Dietary Fiber: 2 g; Protein: 4 g; Cholesterol: 0 mg; Sodium: 1066 mg; Sugars: trace

92. Minty Cucumber Popsicles

Yield: 3 Servings

Total Time: 10 Minutes + Freezing Time

Prep Time: 10 Minutes

Cook Time: N/A

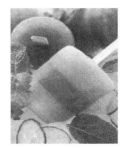

Ingredients:

- 1 cucumber, spirallized
- ¾ cup lime juice, freshly squeezed
- 4 tbsp. fresh mint, chopped
- Water

Directions:

1. Prepare 6 Popsicle molds and in each, place 2 teaspoons of the chopped mint followed by 2 tablespoons of lime juice.

2. Add 2-3 tablespoons of the noodles and top with a bit of water and secure the mold.

3. Freeze the popsicles for a minimum of 4 hours but preferably overnight.

4. Before indulging in your Popsicle, run the mold under some warm water first.

Enjoy!

Nutritional Information per Serving:

Calories: 165; Total Fat: 0.9 g; Carbs: 12.4 g; Dietary Fiber: 3.7 g; Sugars: 9.3 g; Protein: 5.8 g; Cholesterol: 0 mg; Sodium: 32 mg

The Dessert and Drink Recipes

93. Green Tea Avocado Shake

Yield: 2 Servings

Total Time: 5 Minutes

Prep Time: 5 Minutes

Cook Time: N/A

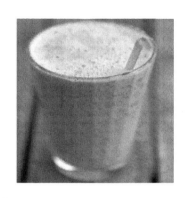

Ingredients

- 1 teaspoon matcha green tea powder
- 1/2 medium avocado
- 1/4 cup vanilla protein powder
- 2 teaspoon liquid stevia
- 2 cups unsweetened almond milk

Directions

Blend all ingredients together until smooth. Enjoy!

Nutritional Information per Serving:

Calories: 172; Total Fat: 13.9 g; Carbs: 7.3 g; Dietary Fiber: 5.4 g; Sugars: 0.6 g; Protein: 6.7 g; Cholesterol: 17 mg; Sodium: 196 mg

94. Berry Power Shake

Yield: 2 Servings

Total Time: 5 Minutes

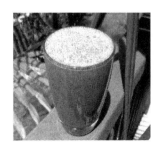

Prep Time: 5 Minutes

Cook Time: N/A

Ingredients

- ¾ cup mixed berries
- 1 cup almond milk
- 1 tbsp. all-natural peanut butter
- 1 tbsp. protein powder
- ¼ tsp. cinnamon powder
- ¼ tsp. ginger, minced

Directions

Place all the ingredients in a blender and mix until smooth.

Nutritional Information per Serving:

Calories: 319; Total Fat: 15 g; Carbs: 9 g; Dietary Fiber: 7.1 g; Sugars: 1.6 g; Protein: 28 g; Cholesterol: 0 mg; Sodium: 93 mg

95. Superfood Chia Pudding

Yield: 1 Serving

Total Time: 5 Minutes

Prep Time: 5 Minutes

Cook Time: N/A

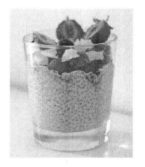

Ingredients

- 25g frozen berries

- 1tbsp chia seeds
- 1 scoop Vanilla protein powder
- 1/2 cup unsweetened almond milk
- Stevia or cocoa, for serving, optional

Directions

Combine all the ingredients in a large bowl; refrigerate for at least 6 hours before serving.

Mix all the ingredients together and put in the fridge overnight or at least a good 6 hours.

96. Healthy Berry Ice Cream

Yield: 4 Servings

Total Time: 10 Minutes

Prep Time: 10 Minutes

Cook Time: N/A

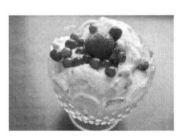

Ingredients

- 500g frozen strawberries, unsweetened
- 420 ml coconut milk
- ½ tbsp. freshly squeezed lemon juice
- 1/tsp stevia extract

Directions

1. Combine all the ingredients in your food processor and pulse until the strawberries are smooth.

2. You can eat it instantly otherwise if you want to eat it later, freeze but take it out 30 minutes before eating because it will be frozen rock-hard due to the lack of sugar.

Enjoy!

Nutritional Information per Serving:

Calories: 201; Total Fat: 7.2 g; Carbs: 19.1 g; Dietary Fiber: 9.2 g; Sugars: 14.3 g; Protein: 6.8 g; Cholesterol: 0 mg; Sodium: 19 mg

97. Delicious Berry Smoothie

Yields: 4 Servings

Total Time: 5 Minutes

Prep Time: 5 Minutes

Cook Time: N/A

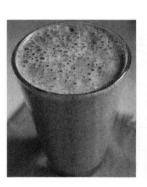

Ingredients:

- 2 cups plain low-fat Greek yogurt
- 1 tablespoon flaxseed
- 2 tablespoons almond butter
- 1 cup frozen blueberries
- 1 cup frozen strawberries
- 1 frozen banana

Directions:

Combine all ingredients in a blender and blend until smooth.

Nutritional Information per Serving:

Calories: 205; Total Fat: 7.6 g; Carbs: 17.7 g; Dietary Fiber: 3.2 g; Protein: 14 g; Cholesterol: 6 mg; Sodium: 38 mg; Sugars: 14 g

98. Delicious Strawberry Punch

Serving Total: 9 servings

Total Time: 5 Minutes

Prep Time: 5 Minutes

Cook Time: N/A

Ingredients:

- 1 cup fresh strawberries
- 4 cups diet ginger ale
- 4 cups fresh pineapple juice

Directions:

Blend the strawberries until smooth. Add ginger ale and pineapple juice and chill for at least 24 hours. Garnish with lime or lemon wedges, if desired.

Nutritional Information per Serving:

Calories: 63; Total Fat: 0.1 g; Carbs: 16 g; Dietary Fiber: trace; Protein: 0.6 g; Cholesterol: 0 mg; Sodium: 8 mg; sugars: 12.1 g

99. Almond-Strawberry Smoothie

Yield: 2-3 Servings

Total Time: 10 Minutes

Prep Time: 10 Minutes

Cook Time: N/A

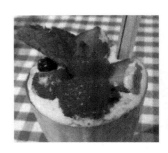

Ingredients

- 500ml almond milk, unsweetened
- ¼ cup frozen strawberries, unsweetened
- 1 scoop vegetarian protein powder
- 100ml heavy cream
- Stevia, to taste

Directions

Combine all the ingredients in a blender and process until smooth.

Serve immediately.

Nutritional Information per Serving:

Calories: 304; Total Fat: 25 g; Carbs: 7 g; Dietary Fiber: 2.5 g; Sugars: 3.9 g; Protein: 15 g; Cholesterol: 71 mg; Sodium: 107 mg

100. Coconut- Coffee smoothie

Yield: 2 Servings

Total Time: 2 Hours

Prep Time: 2 Hours

Cook Time: N/A

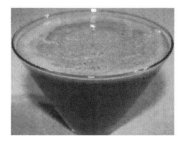

Ingredients

- 2 cups coconut milk, unsweetened
- ½ tsp. cacao powder
- 1-2 drops coconut extract
- 2 tsp. instant coffee
- 2 scoops vanilla protein powder
- Stevia, to taste

Directions

1. Combine all the ingredients in a large measuring cup and stir well to combine. Doesn't have to be super smooth.

2. Transfer to a freezer safe bowl and stir the mixture every 30 minutes.

3. Once frozen, remove from freezer and let stand for about 15 minutes and transfer to the blender and process to a frappe.

Enjoy!

Nutritional Information per Serving:

Calories: 190; Total Fat: 10.3 g; Carbs: 15.8 g; Dietary Fiber: 1.5 g; Sugars: 12.9 g; Protein: 20.7 g; Cholesterol: 0 mg; Sodium: 109 mg

101. Citrus Punch

Serving Total: 2 servings

Total Time: 5 Minutes

Prep Time: 5 Minutes

Cook Time: N/A

Ingredients:

- 1 cup fresh chopped pineapple
- 1/2 cup freshly squeezed lemon juice
- 3 cups water
- 1 cup limeade, frozen

Directions:

1. In a food processor, puree fresh pineapple.

2. Combine the pureed pineapple with the remaining ingredients and chill for at least 1 hour.

Nutritional Information per Serving:

Calories: 54; Total Fat: 0.6 g; Carbs: 12 g; Dietary Fiber: trace; Protein: 0.9 g; Cholesterol: 0 mg; Sodium: 30 mg; sugars: 9.2 g

102. Gingery Lemonade

Serving Total: 4 servings

Total Time: 12 Minutes

Prep Time: 5 Minutes

Cook Time: 7 Minutes

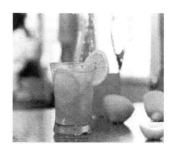

Ingredients:

- 14 slices fresh ginger root
- 4 quarts water
- 1 tablespoon raw honey
- 4 cups fresh lemon juice
- 2 lemons, sliced

Directions:

1. Combine ginger root, water and honey in a saucepan set over medium heat; bring to a gentle boil.

2. Remove from heat and stir in lemon juice. Let cool for about 15 minutes and chill for at least 1 hour.

3. Serve over ice garnished with lemon slices.

Nutritional Information per Serving:

Calories: 98; Total Fat: 2.1 g; Carbs: 10.2 g; Dietary Fiber: 1.1 g; Protein: 2.1 g; Cholesterol: 0 mg; Sodium: 76 mg; sugars: 9.4 g

103. Berry-Spinach Smoothie

Yield: 3 Servings

Total Time: 7 Minutes

Prep Time: 7 Minutes

Cook Time: N/A

Ingredients

- ½ cup reduced fat, plain Greek yogurt
- 1 cup baby spinach
- ¼ cup frozen blueberries, unsweetened
- 1/3 cup almond milk, unsweetened
- 1 scoop vanilla protein powder
- ¼ cup ice

Directions

Combine all the ingredients in a blender and process until smooth or desired consistency is achieved.

Nutritional Information per Serving:

Calories: 270; Total Fat: 13.5 g; Carbs: 6.3 g; Dietary Fiber: 3.5 g; Sugars: 1.9 g; Protein: 11 g; Cholesterol: 0 mg; Sodium: 98 mg

104. Lime Lemon Slush

Serving Total: 2 servings

Total Time: 5 Minutes

Prep Time: 5 Minutes

Cook Time: N/A

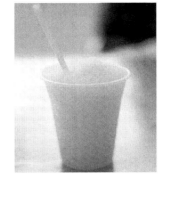

Ingredients:

- 2 limes
- 2 lemons
- 1/8 cup raw honey
- 1 cup pure water
- Ice

Directions:

Blend everything in a blender until smooth. Enjoy!

Nutritional Information per Serving:

Calories: 64; Total Fat: 0 g; Carbs: 17.5 g; Dietary Fiber: trace; Protein: 2.1 g; Cholesterol: 0 mg; Sodium: 2 mg; sugars: 17.4 g

105. Slimming Smoothie

Serving Total: 4 servings

Total Time: 5 Minutes

Prep Time: 5 Minutes

Cook Time: N/A

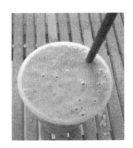

Ingredients:

- 1 ripe avocado
- 1/4 cantaloupe, juiced
- 1 peeled kiwi fruit, juiced

Directions:

Combine the juice and avocado in a blender and blend until smooth.

Nutritional Information per Serving:

Calories: 117; Total Fat: 9.9 g; Carbs: 7.8 g; Dietary Fiber: 4 g; Protein: 1.2 g; Cholesterol: 0 mg; Sodium: 5 mg; sugars: 2.6 g

106. **Gingery Grape Juice**

Serving Total: 1 servings

Total Time: 5 Minutes

Prep Time: 5 Minutes

Cook Time: N/A

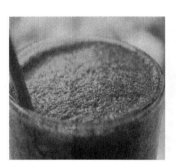

Ingredients:

- 2 cups red grapes
- 1 2-inch peeled ginger
- 1 medium lemon, peeled, juiced
- 4 oz. water

Directions:

Combine all ingredients in a blender; blend until very smooth. Enjoy!

Nutritional Information per Serving:

Calories: 159; Total Fat: 1.1 g; Carbs: 18.8 g; Dietary Fiber: 4 g; Protein: 2.3 g; Cholesterol: 0 mg; Sodium: 10 mg; sugars: 31.5 g

107. Fat-Burner Juice

Yield: 3 Servings

Total Time: 10 Minutes

Prep Time: 10 Minutes

Cook Time: N/A

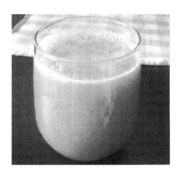

Ingredients

- 1 cup of choice greens
- 2 celery stalks
- 2 green apples
- 2 carrots
- 1 red sweet pepper
- 1 peeled lemon
- 1 ginger

Directions

Juice everything together. Enjoy!

Nutritional Information per Serving:

Calories: 57; Total Fat: 0.2 g; Carbs: 10.7 g; Dietary Fiber: 3.9 g; Protein: 1.7 g; Cholesterol: 0 mg; Sodium: 25 mg; sugars: 8.4 g

108. Garlicky Green Juice

Yield: 2 Servings

Total Time: 10 Minutes

Prep Time: 10 Minutes

Cook Time: N/A

Ingredients

- 1 green apple
- 1 cup kale
- 1 celery stalk
- 1 clove garlic
- Ginger

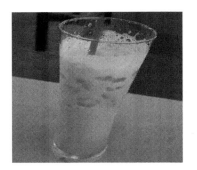

Directions

Juice everything together. Enjoy!

Nutritional Information per Serving:

Calories: 67; Total Fat: 0.2 g; Carbs: 16.8 g; Dietary Fiber: 2.9 g; Protein: 1.2 g; Cholesterol: 0 mg; Sodium: 22 mg; sugars: 9.6 g

109. Strawberry Coconut Milk Smoothie

Yield: 2 Servings

Total me: 5 Minutes

Prep Time: 5 Minutes

Ingredients

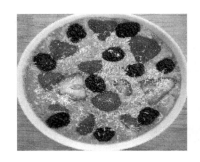

- 2 tbsp. smooth almond butter
- 1 cup coconut milk
- 1 cup frozen strawberries
- 1 scoop protein powder
- 2 packets stevia

Directions

In a blender, combine all ingredients; blend until very smooth. Enjoy!

Nutritional Information per Serving:

Calories: 52; Total Fat: 2.5 g; Carbs: 6.8 g; Dietary Fiber: 4.5 g; Sugars: 1.8 g; Protein: 21.3 g; Cholesterol: 0 mg; Sodium: 72 mg

110. Avocado-Raspberry Smoothie

Yield: 2 Servings

Total me: 5 Minutes

Prep Time: 5 Minutes

Cook Time: N/A

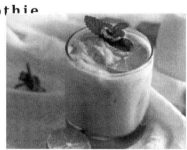

Ingredients
- 1/2 cup frozen raspberries
- ¾ ripe avocado, diced
- 3 tbsp. fresh lemon juice
- 5 drops liquid stevia
- 1 1/3 cup water
- 1 scoop vanilla protein powder

Directions

In a blender, combine all ingredients; blend until very smooth. Enjoy!

Nutritional Information per Serving:
Calories: 227; Total Fat: 20 g; Carbs: 6.4 g; Dietary Fiber: 4.1 g; Sugars: 1.3 g; Protein: 22.6 g; Cholesterol: 0 mg; Sodium: 86 mg

111. Healthy Green Smoothie

Yield: 1 Serving

Total Time: 5 Minutes

Prep Time: 5 Minutes

Cook Time: N/A

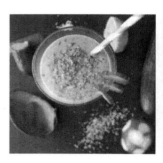

Ingredients
- ½ cup coconut milk
- ½ cup chopped spinach
- ½ medium avocado, diced
- 1 tbsp. extra virgin coconut oil
- ½ tsp. vanilla powder
- ½ cup water
- Handful of ice cubes
- ¼ cup chocolate whey protein
- 1 tsp. matcha powder
- 5 drops liquid stevia

Directions
In a blender, combine all ingredients; blend until very smooth. Enjoy!

Nutritional Information per Serving:

Calories: 468; Total Fat: 48.3 g; Carbs: 6 g; Dietary Fiber: 4.5 g; Sugars: 1.2 g; Protein: 14.2 g; Cholesterol: 0 mg; Sodium: 109 mg

112. The Super-8 Detox Juice

Yield: 2 Servings

Total Time: 10 Minutes

Prep Time: 10 Minutes

Cook Time: N/A

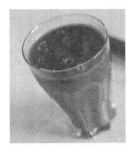

Ingredients

- 1 collard leaf
- 1 kale leaf
- 1 broccoli floret
- 1 tomato
- 1/2 red pepper
- 1 carrot
- 1 stalk of celery
- Handful of parsley

Directions

Juice all ingredients and enjoy!

Nutritional Information per Serving:

Calories: 66; Total Fat: 0.4 g; Carbs: 13.8 g; Dietary Fiber: 4.2 g; Protein: 3.6 g; Cholesterol: 0 mg; Sodium: 64 mg; sugars: 4.5 g

113. Sugar-Free Peanut Butter Protein Smoothie

Yield: 2 Servings

Total Time: 2 Minutes

Prep Time: 2 Minutes

Cook Time: N/A

Ingredients

- 1 tablespoon natural peanut butter
- 1/2 cup low-fat cottage cheese
- 1/2 cup unsweetened almond milk
- 1 scoop Whey Protein
- 2 drops liquid stevia
- 1 cup ice cubes
- Drizzle of peanut butter and cacao nibs
- Pinch of chicory powder

Directions

In a blender, blend together peanut butter, cottage cheese, almond milk, whey protein, stevia and ice until very smooth. Serve over ice drizzled with peanut butter and sprinkled with cacao nibs and chicory powder.

Nutritional Information per Serving:

Calories: 187; Total Fat: 8.2 g; Carbs: 6.4 g; Dietary Fiber: 0.9 g; Sugars: 7.1 g; Protein: 21.4 g; Cholesterol: 37 mg; Sodium: 319 mg

114. Kale-Beetroot Juice

Yield: 1 Serving

Total Time: 5 Minutes

Prep Time: 5 Minutes

Cook Time: N/A

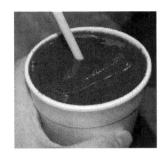

Ingredients

- 2 leaves of Kale
- 1 apple, cored
- 2 carrots, chopped
- 1 stalk of celery, chopped
- 1 small beetroot, chopped

Directions

Combine all the ingredients together in a blender and blend until smooth.

Nutritional Information per Serving:

Calories: 201; Total Fat: 0.5 g; Carbs: 19.6 g; Dietary Fiber: 9.9 g; Protein: 4 g; Cholesterol: 0 mg; Sodium: 179 mg; sugars: 31.9 g

115. Ginger Spice Smoothie

Yield: 1 Serving

Total Time: 5 Minutes

Prep Time: 5 Minutes

Cook Time: N/A

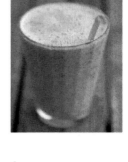

Ingredients

- 1 nub ginger root, finely minced
- 1 cup chopped spinach
- 1 tsp. Cinnamon
- 1 cup Purified Water
- 1 scoop protein powder

Directions

Combine together all the ingredients in a blender and blend until very smooth. Enjoy!

Nutritional Information per Serving:

Calories: 53; Total Fat: 0.1 g; Carbs: 4.9 g; Dietary Fiber: 3.4 g; Sugars: 1.1 g; Protein: 19.7 g; Cholesterol: 0 mg; Sodium: 95 mg

116. Lemon Blueberry Bliss

Yields: 2 Servings

Total Time: 5 Minutes

Prep Time: 5 Minutes

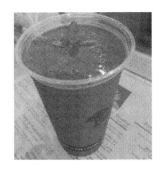

Ingredients:

- 2 cups frozen blueberries
- 1 cup organic baby spinach
- 1 pear, halved and cored
- 1 cup coconut water
- 2 tbsp. freshly squeezed lemon juice
- 1 tsp. freshly grated lemon zest
- 1 scoop protein powder

Directions:

Add all the ingredients to a blender and blend to your desired consistency. Enjoy!

Nutritional Information per Serving:

Calories: 156; Total Fat: 1 g; Carbs: 6 g; Dietary Fiber: 4.5 g; Sugars: 1.9 g; Protein: 12.3 g; Cholesterol: 0 mg; Sodium: 231 mg

117. Yummy Cinnamon Smoothie

Yield: 2 Servings

Total Time: 7 Minutes

Prep Time: 7 Minutes

Cook Time: N/A

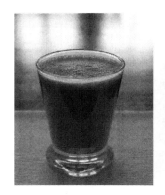

Ingredients

- 1 cup almond milk, unsweetened
- ½ tsp ground cinnamon
- 1 tsp flax meal
- 2 tbsp. vanilla protein powder
- ¼ tsp pure vanilla extract
- Stevia, to taste
- ½ -1 cup ice

Directions

Combine all the ingredients in a blender and process until creamy, smooth and thick

Serve immediately.

Nutritional Information per Serving:

Calories: 145; Total Fat: 3.2 g; Carbs: 1.6 g; Dietary Fiber: 0.5 g; Sugars: 0.9 g; Protein: 26 g; Cholesterol: 0 mg; Sodium: 79 mg

118. Mint-Infused Green Smoothie

Yield: 2 Servings

Total Time: 5 Minutes

Prep Time: 5 Minutes

Cook Time: N/A

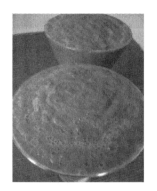

Ingredients

- 1 cup fresh baby spinach
- ½ an avocado
- ½ cup almond milk, unsweetened
- ¼ tsp peppermint extract
- 1 scoop vegetarian protein powder
- 3/4 cup ice
- Stevia, to taste
- Cacao nibs, optional

Directions

Blend all the ingredients until smooth and thick.

Serve immediately!

Nutritional Information per Serving:

Calories: 220; Total Fat: 13.3 g; Carbs: 5.8 g; Dietary Fiber: 1.5 g; Sugars: 2.9 g; Protein: 20.7 g; Cholesterol: 0 mg; Sodium: 102 mg

119. Gingery Pineapple Paradise

Yield: 2 Servings

Total Time: 5 Minutes

Prep Time: 5 Minutes

Cook Time: N/A

Ingredients

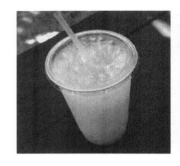

- 1-inch piece fresh ginger
- 1/2 cup pineapple chunks
- 2 tablespoons lime juice
- 1 apple, diced
- 1/2 cup mango chunks

Directions

Blend together all ingredients until smooth. Serve over ice.

Nutritional Information per Serving:

Calories: 186; Total Fat: 0.8 g; Carbs: 17.2 g; Dietary Fiber: 6.6 g; Protein: 1.8 g; Cholesterol: 0 mg; Sodium: 6 mg; sugars: 28.7 g

120. Toasted Coconut & Strawberry Smoothie

Yields: 1 Servings

Total Time: 15 Minutes

Prep Time: 10 Minutes

Cook Time: 5 Minutes

Ingredients:

- 1 tbsp. freshly squeezed lemon juice
- 2 cups frozen strawberries
- 2 cups coconut milk (unsweetened)
- 1 tsp. honey
- 1 tbsp. spirulina
- 2 tbsp. toasted coconut shavings, divided

Directions:

1. Combine all the ingredients in a blender and only 1 tablespoon of the toasted coconut shavings; blend until very smooth and creamy.

2. Toast the remaining coconut shavings in the oven at 350°F for about 3 minutes or until golden brown.

3. Serve the smoothie in four tall serving glasses and top each with the toasted coconut.

Nutritional Information Per Serving:

Calories: 81; Total Fat: 4 g; Total Carb: 10 g; Protein: 2 g; Dietary fiber: 3 g

Made in the USA
San Bernardino, CA
04 April 2018